SLOW COOKER DOG FOOD COOKBOOK

The Ultimate Guide to Vet-Endorsed, Quick & Easy Homemade Recipes – Affordable, Nutritious Meals for Busy Owners, Ensuring Lifelong Health & Joy for Dogs of All Breeds

MORGAN J. NICHOLS

Table of Contents

Preface

Hello, fellow dog-lovers!

Welcome to the *Slow Cooker Dog Food Cookbook*. My name is Morgan J. Nichols, and I'm thrilled to be guiding you on this path to provide the greatest nutrition for your pet.

Growing up in the beautiful town of Bar Harbor, Maine, dogs were always a part of my life, whether as playful puppies or loyal companions. However, it was my energetic Labrador, Alex, who introduced me to the realm of canine nutrition. During a difficult period marked by work stress and family obligations, Alex's steadfast support served as my anchor. When he started to show signs of exhaustion and his once-shiny coat turned dull, I realized something was wrong. The commercial food I trusted may not have provided him with the necessary nutrients.

I was eager to find a solution, so I started researching and testing. That's when I realized how beneficial slow cooking can be for dogs. Slow-cooked food retains more nutrients and flavor, making it healthier and more enticing to our canine companions. Moreover, this cooking method worked perfectly with my hectic schedule, allowing me to create nutritious meals for Alex without spending hours in the kitchen.

Over time, my kitchen transformed into a mini-test lab where neighbors, friends, and dog owners excitedly tested my culinary experiments. Responses were very positive, and dogs with a wide range of health problems, from allergies to stomach problems, showed big improvements. Requests for recipes and meal plans began to flood in, consequently driving me to hone my approach. I've attended multiple courses and spoken with experienced doctors to ensure that my recipes are both nutritious and effective, solidifying my authority in canine nutrition beyond that of a hobbyist.

Inspired by these changes and growing community interest, I set out to build a comprehensive guide to canine nutrition rather than just a recipe collection. My objective is to provide you with the knowledge and skills you need to give your dogs the best care possible. This book contains well-tested, vet-endorsed recipes that address the dietary demands of various canines. Indeed, everyone, whether they are a joyful puppy, an active adult, or an aging dog, will find something to enjoy.

I designed each recipe in this book to be simple and easy to prepare, even if you have no cooking experience. Using inexpensive, easy-to-find items enables you to feed your pets healthy, handmade meals without breaking the bank or spending too much time in the kitchen. Our emphasis on practicality and convenience therefore allows even the busiest dog owners to feed their pups balanced diets.

Slow Cooker Dog Food Cookbook also addresses prevalent worries by providing practical counsel and soothing recommendations. I understand how scary transitioning to home-made dog food can be, but don't worry. From quantity management and nutritional requirements to meal planning and time-saving strategies, you'll find everything you need to provide the best care for your dog.

There is nothing more fulfilling than seeing your dog happy and healthy as a result of your kitchen efforts. This journey is about more than simply food; it's about love, care, and the long-term satisfaction that comes from giving your pet the finest. That being said, I appreciate your trust in me to lead you through this process. I truly hope you make the best use of this book.

Warmest regards.

Morgan J. Nichols

Introduction
Welcome to the World of Homemade Dog Food!

Welcome to a new era in which the health and happiness of our beloved dogs take center stage. Ever wondered what ingredients are in store-bought kibble? Devoted owners seeking the best for their dogs have been asking this question, and they are increasingly taking the popularity of homemade dog food beyond the mere trend. Rising awareness of the ingredients in commercial dog food and a desire to provide healthier, more natural options are driving this shift toward homemade meals.

Many dog owners have been wondering about the ingredients in store-bought kibble, which has led to an increase in the popularity of preparing nutritious and enjoyable homemade meals.

Homemade dog food provides various advantages. Firstly, it allows you complete control over the ingredients, ensuring that your dog receives high-quality proteins, healthy fats, and a well-balanced diet of vitamins and minerals. Forget about the hidden ingredients, preservatives, and low-quality fillers found in commercial dog food. Whether your dog has allergies, sensitivities, or a picky palate, you can customize every meal to meet their exact nutritional requirements.

Making homemade dog food can also save money and time, particularly when using a slow cooker. Slow cooking retains the nutritional value of the ingredients, ensuring that your dog gets the most out of each meal. It's a simple, stress-free approach to ensuring your dog's meals are both nutritious and tasty. Imagine the perfume of fresh chicken and vegetables boiling in your kitchen, filling the air with a fragrance that will make your human family members envy you.

A greater understanding of canine nutrition is additionally driving the trend toward homemade dog food. Websites such as *PetMD* and the *American Kennel Club (AKC)* offer helpful materials and guidelines to help pet owners make informed decisions about their dogs' meals. These materials simplify the process of properly feeding your dog, from critical nutrients to portion control. It's more than just filling a bowl; it's about feeding your dog in a way that promotes general health, longevity, and happiness.

Another motivating element behind this movement is the emotional bond we have with our pets. Dogs are more than simply pets; they are part of the family. Therefore, like any other family member, they deserve the highest level of care. There's a huge joy in knowing that you're helping your dog's well-being with each meal you prepare. Cooking for your dog is an act of love that strengthens your bond with them, transforming mealtime into a shared experience of affection and care.

Feedback from dog owners who have switched to homemade food has been quite encouraging. There are countless stories of dogs with brighter coats, higher energy, and better digestion. For example, Laura described how her Labrador, Bella, transformed after switching to homemade meals, becoming more lively and vivacious. Such testimonies underscore the concrete benefits of homemade dog food, motivating more pet owners to take the leap.

As you embark on this path of producing homemade dog food, keep in mind that the goal is not perfection but rather making a positive impact. Whether you're a seasoned cook or a beginner in the kitchen, there's a dish for you and your dog. Together, we can make sure our dogs have healthier, happier lives, one slow-cooked meal at a time.

Chapter 1
Understanding Dog Nutrition

Essential Nutrients for Dogs

Proteins are essential in a dog's diet because they help build muscle and maintain general bodily function. Lean meats such as chicken, beef, and fish, as well as plant-based choices like lentils and chickpeas, are excellent sources of protein. These proteins contain important amino acids, which are required for tissue repair and immune function.

Fats provide a concentrated supply of energy for your dog's metabolic functions. Essential fatty acids, notably Omega-3 and Omega-6, are critical for maintaining a healthy coat, decreasing inflammation, and enhancing cognitive function. Fish oil, flaxseed oil, and coconut oil are all good sources of these healthy fats. Moreover, including healthy fats in your dog's diet provides energy for everyday activities and aids in the absorption of fat-soluble vitamins.

Vitamins and minerals serve critical roles in many biological activities. Vitamins A, D, E, K, C, and B-complex are vital for a dog's health. For instance, Vitamin A promotes vision and immunological function, while vitamin D is essential for calcium absorption and bone health. Acting as an antioxidant, vitamin E prevents harm to cells, whereas vitamin K is required for blood clotting. Vitamin C promotes immunological function and collagen formation, and B-complex vitamins help in energy metabolism. Minerals like calcium, phosphorus, and magnesium help with bone strength, muscular function, and nerve transmission.

Carbohydrates regulate your dog's blood sugar levels and are necessary for optimal digestive function. Complex carbohydrates present in vegetables, legumes, and whole grains contain dietary fiber, which aids with digestive health. These carbs provide a slow-release energy source, thus keeping your dog active and healthy all day.

Finally, water is the most important nutrient of all. It is required for all metabolic activities in a dog's body, including digestion and temperature regulation. A constant supply of fresh and drinking water for your dog is essential. Dehydration can cause major health problems, so it's critical to watch your dog's water consumption, particularly in hot weather or after heavy activity.

Nutritional Needs by Life Stage

Puppies: Building a Strong Foundation

Feeding pups ensures that they get the right nutrients to sustain their rapid growth and development. Puppies require a protein, fat, vitamin, and mineral-rich diet during their first year of life in order to create strong muscles, promote brain development, and strengthen their immune systems. High-quality proteins, like beef, chicken, and fish, include vital amino acids for growth. A diverse range of protein sources ensures a well-balanced intake of these essential elements.

Fats are essential in a puppy's diet, giving concentrated energy and promoting brain development. Fish oil and flaxseed include omega-3 and omega-6 fatty acids, which help maintain healthy skin and a glossy coat while also improving cognitive function. Puppies require more energy than adult dogs, and fats help supply those demands effectively, driving their energetic antics and endless curiosity.

Additionally, puppies require vitamins and minerals for growth. Calcium and phosphorus are essential for the formation of strong bones and teeth. Leafy greens contain these minerals, which help prevent developmental disorders such as rickets. Vitamins A, D, and E improve vision, immunological function, and overall health. Carrots, sweet potatoes, and spinach are high in these vitamins, making them ideal additions to your puppy's diet.

Carbohydrates give energy for your puppy's everyday activities and promote healthy digestion. Whole grains like oats, brown rice, sweet potatoes, and peas are good carbohydrate sources. These components not only provide long-lasting energy, but they also include fiber, which facilitates digestion and promotes gut health. Fiber is essential for preventing digestive disorders such as constipation and keeping your puppy's digestive tract running normally.

Hydration is also an important part of puppy feeding. Always make sure your puppy has access to fresh, clean water, particularly in the case of dry-food eaters. Proper hydration supports all biological functions, including digestion and temperature regulation.

Furthermore, feeding frequency is a significant aspect. Puppies often require more frequent feedings than adult dogs to maintain energy levels and stimulate growth. Starting with four meals per day and progressively reducing to two as they get older helps prevent problems such as hypoglycemia, which pups are prone to because of their quick metabolism and small stomachs.

Using a slow cooker to make dog food might be especially useful. Slow cooking retains the nutritional integrity of the ingredients, ensuring that your puppy benefits the most from each meal. The gentle cooking process makes proteins, vitamins, and minerals more accessible, which means they are easier for your puppy to absorb and use.

Adults: Maintaining Health and Vitality

Adult dogs require a well-balanced diet that contains high-quality proteins, carbs, healthy fats, vitamins, and minerals. Proteins remain essential for muscle maintenance and repair. Lean meats such as beef, chicken, and fish are high in amino acids that adult dogs require for robust muscles and tissues. Furthermore, to avoid gastrointestinal difficulties, ensure that these proteins are easily digestible.

Fats are also important for adult dogs, as they provide concentrated energy. Healthy fats, such as those found in fish oil, flaxseed oil, and coconut oil, help cells function, improve fat-soluble vitamin absorption, and maintain a lustrous coat and healthy skin. Omega-3 and omega-6 fatty acids, in particular, play important roles in decreasing inflammation and improving heart function. Including these fats in your dog's diet can help to keep their energy levels consistent and their overall health under control.

Carbohydrates supply energy and are essential for a healthy digestive tract. Whole grains, such as brown rice and oats, as well as vegetables like sweet potatoes and carrots, are beneficial sources of carbohydrates. They not only provide energy, but they also contain fiber, which is necessary for digestive health. Fiber regulates bowel motions and can prevent constipation and diarrhea, ensuring your dog's digestive tract runs properly.

Moreover, vitamins and minerals are the hidden heroes of your dog's diet. Vitamins A, D, E, and K serve vital roles in a variety of biological activities, including vision and immunological support. Calcium, phosphorus, and potassium are necessary minerals for bone and tooth strength, neuron function, and muscular contraction. Incorporating a variety of vegetables and fruits, such as spinach, carrots, and blueberries, can help meet your dog's nutritional needs organically, delivering a wide range of nutrients.

You should tailor an adult dog's diet to their breed, health status, and activity level. For instance, more active dogs may require a larger calorie intake, whereas less active or elderly dogs may require fewer calories to avoid weight gain. Regular vet check-ups can help you customize your dog's diet to their specific needs, ensuring they get the appropriate balance of nutrients.

Hydration is also an important part of an adult dog's diet. Fresh, clean water should always be accessible to help your dog's digestion and overall health, especially if he eats dry food. Proper hydration promotes organ function and prevents dehydration, which can cause major health problems.

Using a slow cooker to prepare your dog's food is a fantastic way to make sure they receive a well-balanced diet. The smell of slow-cooked food can make feeding time more pleasant for your dog, increasing their appetite and satisfaction.

Seniors: Supporting Aging Bodies

As dogs age, their nutritional demands fluctuate dramatically to match changes in their bodies and overall health. Feeding a senior dog involves a thorough awareness of their changing needs in order to keep them healthy and comfortable. Proteins are still important for elderly dogs, but the emphasis should shift to easily digestible, high-quality options. Aging dogs can lose muscle mass; therefore, consuming lean meats such as chicken, turkey, and fish can aid with muscle maintenance and repair. Supplement these proteins with an adequate quantity of fat to prevent excessive weight gain, which can exacerbate joint difficulties and other age-related concerns.

Fats remain an important part of a senior dog's diet, but the type and amount must be carefully considered. Healthy fats, such as Omega-3 and Omega-6 fatty acids found in fish oil and flaxseed, promote brain function and reduce inflammation, which is especially beneficial for dogs suffering from arthritis or other inflammatory disorders. Consuming these fats in moderation promotes a lustrous coat and healthy skin while also improving overall cognitive function.

Carbohydrates from high-fiber sources can help improve digestion and blood sugar levels. Whole grains, such as sweet potatoes, brown rice, and oats, are wonderful options. Fiber is crucial for senior dogs because it encourages healthy bowel movements and can avoid constipation, which is a typical problem in older canines. These carbs provide a constant release of energy, keeping your senior dog energetic and engaged all day.

Senior dogs need vitamins and minerals to stay in good health. Antioxidant-rich foods, such as blueberries and spinach, might be useful in lowering oxidative stress and increasing immunity. Calcium and phosphorus are essential for maintaining bone density and avoiding osteoporosis, which can be a problem in older dogs. Incorporating leafy greens and fortified ingredients ensures that older dogs get enough vitamins and minerals to maintain their overall health and well-being.

Hydration is another important part of a senior dog's diet. Older dogs are more prone to dehydration, so provide a constant supply of clean and fresh water for them. Wet foods, or adding water to dry kibble, can also help them drink more water, which promotes better kidney function and general hydration.

Feeding frequency and portion control become increasingly critical as dogs age. Senior dogs benefit from more frequent, smaller meals, which can aid digestion and minimize weight gain. Monitoring their weight and modifying portions properly is critical for avoiding obesity, which can lead to additional health concerns.

Slow cookers can be extremely useful for preparing meals for senior pets. The slow cooking procedure helps to break down components, making them more digestible and gentler on an older dog's stomach. It also enables the incorporation of diverse, nutrient-dense foods in a way that improves their flavor and palatability, guaranteeing that even the pickiest senior dog enjoys their meals. This deliberate approach to nutrition promotes physical health, cognitive function, and overall well-being, ensuring that their older years are as enjoyable and satisfying as possible.

Safe Ingredients for Dogs

Making nutritious homemade dog food begins with choosing safe and helpful components. Proteins are essential, and selecting healthy sources of animal protein such as beef, turkey, chicken, and fish is critical. These meats contain necessary amino acids that aid in muscle building, tissue repair, and immunological function. Incorporating a variety of protein sources can help to reduce nutritional monotony and provide your dog with a diverse range of nutrients.

Fruits and vegetables supply critical vitamins, minerals, and fiber for your dog's diet. Apples (seedless), blueberries, carrots, spinach, and sweet potatoes are all safe and nutritious selections. Each fruit and vegetable has its own nutrient profile; for example, apples contain vitamins A and C, but carrots high in beta-carotene promote eye health. Blueberries are high in antioxidants, spinach has iron and magnesium, and sweet potatoes include fiber as well as vitamins A and C. These nutrient-dense foods improve your dog's general health and contribute to a well-balanced diet.

If you use grains and legumes properly, you can safely include them in your dog's diet. Brown rice, quinoa, and lentils are excellent options. These grains and legumes have complex carbohydrates that provide long-lasting energy and improve intestinal health. Fiber in these components helps to regulate bowel motions and keep the gut healthier. Balancing fiber and carbohydrate consumption keeps your dog active and prevents stomach disorders.

Fats and oils are essential for a glossy, healthy coat and overall well-being. Fish oil and flaxseed oil, both high in Omega-3 fatty acids, as well as coconut oil, which contains medium-chain triglycerides, are safe sources of healthy fats. These oils promote skin health, decrease inflammation, and improve cognitive function. Including a range of fats in your dog's diet promotes the uptake of fat-soluble vitamins and provides an effective source of energy.

Herbs and spices can be healthy if used in moderation. Safe herbs and spices, like basil, parsley, and turmeric, not only improve flavor but also provide health advantages. People recognize parsley for its breath-freshening benefits and high vitamin C content, turmeric for its anti-inflammatory characteristics, and basil for its antioxidants that can aid in stress alleviation. Including these in your dog's food can improve palatability and general health.

Ensuring the nutritional value and efficacy of these substances is critical to maintaining your dog's health and lifespan. This holistic approach to dog feeding not only meets their nutritional requirements but also improves their quality of life.

Foods to Avoid

On the other hand, knowing which foods to avoid is critical for their safety and wellness. Certain compounds that are healthy and useful for humans might be toxic or even lethal to dogs. One of the best-known examples is chocolate, which contains theobromine. Dogs absorb theobromine slowly, which causes symptoms such as vomiting, diarrhea, rapid breathing, an elevated heart rate, and seizures. This substance is particularly hazardous in dark chocolate and baking chocolate.

Grapes and raisins are also extremely poisonous to dogs, resulting in renal failure even in small quantities. Symptoms include vomiting, tiredness, and decreased appetite, which can result in long-term kidney damage or acute renal failure. Similarly, onions and garlic, whether raw, cooked, or powdered, can harm red blood cells and induce anemia. Anemia in dogs is characterized by weakness, lethargy, and shortness of breath. A small dose may not cause instant harm, but repeated consumption can have a cumulative effect.

Xylitol, a sugar replacement widely found in sugar-free products such as candy, gum, and baked goods, is severely harmful to dogs. Even modest dosages can trigger a fast release of insulin, resulting in hypoglycemia, seizures, liver failure, and even death. If you're feeding your dog or making homemade treats, always check the labels for xylitol. Additionally, you should never give alcohol or alcohol-containing meals to dogs, as even small amounts can cause vomiting, diarrhea, trouble breathing, convulsions, and even death.

Avocados contain persin, which can cause nausea and diarrhea. Although small quantities of avocado might not pose a significant risk, it's advisable to refrain from feeding your dog avocado, especially the pit, skin, and leaves, due to their elevated persin content. Likewise, avoid including macadamia nuts in your dog's diet, as they may lead to symptoms such as weakness, depression, vomiting, tremors, and overheating.

Avoid feeding heated bones to your dog, as they can splinter and cause choking or tearing in the digestive tract. Instead, use raw, meaty bones appropriate for your dog's size and chewing inclinations. Be cautious with fat trimmings as well; while limited amounts of fat are important for a healthy diet, too much can cause pancreatitis, which causes severe pain, vomiting, and dehydration.

Meat, chicken, dairy products, wheat, and soy can contain allergens, which cause itching, ear infections, and gastrointestinal distress. Identifying and avoiding them is critical, and gradually introducing new foods can aid in monitoring for allergic reactions. Other foods, even if they are not harmful or allergic, might induce digestive problems. Fatty and spicy foods, as well as dairy products, might cause stomach distress, diarrhea, and bloating. Managing sensitivities and intolerances necessitates careful observation and the elimination of problematic foods from your dog's diet.

Avoiding dangerous ingredients such as artificial colors, flavors, and preservatives is critical for keeping your dog healthy. Many commercial dog diets contain these ingredients, which can contribute to a variety of health concerns, like allergies or behavioral disorders. Therefore, choose natural alternatives, such as fresh herbs and spices, to provide flavor but also nutritional value.

By becoming aware of these potentially dangerous foods and substances, you can ensure that your dog's diet is both nutritious and safe. This proactive approach to their nutritional needs will help them avoid health problems and improve their general well-being.

Chapter 2
Practicalities of Healthy Home Cooking

Benefits and Real-World Advantages

Switching to homemade dog food has numerous practical benefits for your dog's health and well-being. One significant advantage is the higher nutritional value that handmade meals bring. For instance, when my neighbor converted her allergic dog to a homemade diet, she was able to eliminate common allergens such as chicken and wheat and replace them with turkey and sweet potatoes. This modification significantly improved her dog's skin condition and energy levels, demonstrating the importance of diet for health.

Another real-world advantage is the increased digestion of fresh, high-quality ingredients. Moreover, fresh food is easier for dogs to digest than processed commercial options. For example, my friend found her dog had less bloating and firmer stools after switching to a homemade diet. This change made her dog more comfortable while also making house-keeping easier and simplifying pet ownership.

Customization is one of the most compelling reasons to make homemade dog food. Every dog has different health issues, allergies, and preferences. For instance, I created a diet for a dog with kidney difficulties that included low-phosphorus items such as lean meats and specific veggies. This diet effectively controlled the dog's disease and improved its quality of life.

Cost-effectiveness is another key advantage. Although the initial notion may be that home-made dog food is pricey, a thorough cost analysis frequently finds the contrary. Many pet owners discover that by purchasing ingredients in bulk and taking advantage of seasonal produce, they can feed their dogs high-quality meals at a lower cost than premium com-mercial feeds. For example, a friend who switched to homemade dog food said that her monthly food expenses decreased by 20%, resulting in significant savings for her household.

Increased variety in your dog's diet can help prevent nutritional deficits and make meals more interesting. Unlike kibble, homemade diets allow for the incorporation of a diverse spectrum of foods. This variant guarantees a more complete nutritional intake. For in-stance, rotating different meats and veggies can help your dog avoid boredom while also providing a diverse range of nutrients.

Another benefit of cooking fresh meals is the emotional connection it fosters. Love for your pet can strengthen your bond through food preparation. I recall a lovely anecdote from a fellow dog owner who shared how the act of preparing her dog's meals became a cherished ritual, enhancing their bond.

Switching to homemade food can also help to address difficulties with commercial dog food, such as low-quality fillers and artificial additives. These components frequently con-tribute to long-term health issues. By gradually moving to homemade meals, you may avoid gastric discomfort and ensure your dog's seamless adaptation to the new diet. For example, beginning with a simple chicken and rice recipe and gradually introducing new ingredients can help your dog acclimate without causing any negative reactions.

As a result, relying on high-quality ingredients and specialized recipes can significantly improve your dog's health and well-being, ensuring an enjoyable and healthy life for your beloved companion.

Addressing Common Concerns and Misconceptions

Shifting to homemade dog food might be intimidating, especially given the myriad worries and myths surrounding the procedure. One major worry is the apparent time burden associated with cooking prepared meals. Efficient meal preparation options, such as batch cooking, using a slow cooker, and freezing portions, can therefore drastically minimize the amount of time necessary. For example, my friend Lisa can prepare a week's worth of meals in one afternoon by utilizing a slow cooker and freezing the servings. This allows her to prepare nutritious, fresh meals for her dog, Max, without having to cook them every day.

Moreover, homemade meals must provide a comprehensive and balanced diet, which can be accomplished by conducting extensive research and working with veterinary nutritionists. Regulatory compliance for maintaining dietary balance is another major concern that is critical to ensuring that homemade dog food fulfills established nutritional criteria. Understanding the AAFCO and NRC criteria can help you guarantee that your recipes are nutritionally full and balanced. Regularly checking these guidelines and changing recipes as appropriate will help maintain compliance and guarantee your dog gets the best nutrition.

Additionally, cost is a major worry for many dog owners. While people may believe homemade dog food is pricey, a thorough cost study frequently finds the reverse. Many pet owners discover that by purchasing ingredients in bulk and selecting seasonal produce, they can feed their dogs high-quality meals at a lower cost than premium commercial feeds. To illustrate, my colleague Sarah reported that switching to homemade dog meals reduced her monthly food expenses by 20%.

Safety is frequently questioned, with concerns about nutrient deficits and food safety measures at the forefront. Address these concerns by following conventional food safety recommendations, such as fully washing products, cooking meats to the right temperature, and avoiding cross-contamination. Furthermore, adopting a range of foodstuffs might help prevent shortages because different foods contain different nutrients. For example, alternating between chicken, turkey, and beef results in a more balanced intake of vital nutrients.

The health risks of homemade dog food are widely exaggerated. Myths about homemade diets being hazardous can be debunked by emphasizing scientific research that supports the benefits of eating fresh, whole foods. For instance, research has shown that dogs fed well-balanced homemade foods had better health outcomes than those fed commercial diets. One study found that dogs on homemade food had better fur and greater energy than those on traditional diets.

Understanding dog food labels might be difficult, but it is necessary in order to make conscious decisions. Many commercial dog foods contain misleading information and deceptive marketing practices. Understanding these labels can help you select high-quality items while avoiding those with dangerous ingredients. For example, focusing on the full, natural ingredients indicated on labels will help you select the best food for your dog.

Finally, troubleshooting common challenges with homemade diets entails identifying and treating concerns, including finicky eaters and food intolerances. Experiment with different ingredients, introduce new foods gradually, and make adjustments based on your dog's tastes and health responses. For example, my dog originally refused various vegetables, but after progressively blending them with his favorite dishes, he eventually accepted and appreciated them.

Addressing these frequent worries and misconceptions regarding homemade dog food might help your dog transition smoothly and successfully to a new diet.

Monitor and Maintain Health

Ensuring your dog's health and longevity requires regular monitoring and proactive maintenance of their diet and overall well-being. Regular weight checks and body condition grading are critical for monitoring your dog's health. This method involves feeling your dog's ribs and looking for an evident waistline to assess whether they are underweight, overweight, or at an optimal weight. It is critical that you adjust your dog's diet in response to these observations. For instance, if your dog gains weight, you may need to cut portion sizes or use lower-calorie components.

Digestive health is another important aspect to examine. Additionally, observing stool quality and frequency might provide valuable information about your dog's digestive tract. Healthy stools are usually firm and moist, but variations in quality, color, or frequency may suggest digestive problems or dietary intolerances. Diarrhea, constipation, and extremely soft stools are all signs of poor digestion. Therefore, if you observe these symptoms, you may need to change your diet, add additional fiber, or avoid certain items that are creating problems.

Behavioral changes can indicate your dog's health. Monitoring energy levels, temperament, and behavior is critical. Abrupt reductions in energy, increased irritation, or unusual behaviors may signal nutritional concerns or health problems. Early detection allows for dietary adjustments and veterinary consultation. In addition, keeping your dog active and involved is critical to their physical and emotional well-being.

Long-term health maintenance for your dog requires a balanced diet. This entails reviewing and modifying your dog's food on a regular basis to accommodate changing nutritional needs as they age or increase their level of exercise. For example, elderly dogs may require more joint support from supplements such as glucosamine, while younger, more active dogs may require a greater protein intake to maintain muscle growth.

Implementing these routines not only provides immediate health benefits but also helps to sustain those benefits over time. In conclusion, monitoring and maintaining your dog's health involves setting weight check reminders, keeping a journal of dietary changes and their consequences, and frequently modifying your dog's food plan with the assistance of a veterinary nutritionist.

Chapter 3
Getting Started with Slow Cooking

Why Use a Slow Cooker?

Using a slow cooker to prepare your dog's food has various benefits that address both pet owners' busy lifestyles and their pets' nutritional demands. The main advantage is convenience. With a slow cooker, you can add the necessary ingredients, set the timer, and get on with your day. This hands-off method is ideal for busy operators who wish to deliver homemade meals without devoting hours to the kitchen. Whether you're busy with work, family, or other responsibilities, a slow cooker guarantees that your dog's meals are ready with no effort, making it an excellent alternative for individuals with hectic schedules.

Another significant benefit of slow cooking is that it preserves nutrients. Slow cooking preserves more vitamins and minerals than high-heat cooking methods. Consequently, your dog's meals become healthier due to the mild, sustained heat that prevents the loss of nutrients. Ingredients such as vegetables and lean meats retain their nutritional value, delivering key nutrients such as vitamins, minerals, and antioxidants that are critical for your dog's health. This way of cooking guarantees that each meal contains the most nutritional value, benefiting your dog's general health.

Moreover, slow cooking provides additional benefits, such as improved flavor and digestion. The gradual, steady cooking allows the flavors to blend together, making the meal more appealing to your dog. Slow cooking also breaks down proteins and fibers more effectively than other cooking methods, resulting in more digestible meals for your dog. This might be especially beneficial in order to help dogs who suffer from gastrointestinal issues or sensitivity.

When choosing a slow cooker, evaluate the capacity and size that will best fit your needs. A 6 to 8-quart slow cooker is perfect for large dogs or many pets since it allows you to prepare large batches of food at once, saving time and ensuring you have plenty of meals on hand. A 3- to 4-quart slow cooker may be more suited to smaller dogs or single servings, reducing waste and making storage easier. This size versatility accommodates a variety of needs, ensuring that you always prepare the appropriate amount of food for your pet.

Programmability is an important element of a slow cooker. You can specify specific cooking durations and temperatures with models with programmable settings, guaranteeing perfect cooking every time. This feature is especially handy for busy owners since they can program the slow cooker to begin cooking at a given time, guaranteeing that dinner is ready when they arrive home. Look for a slow cooker with a digital timer and an automatic keep warm function, which keeps the food at the proper temperature until you're ready to serve. This ensures that your dog's food is constantly fresh and ready to eat, even when you are not home.

The material and construction quality of the slow cooker are very crucial. Slow cookers with ceramic or stainless steel components are durable and easy to clean. Ceramic inserts are ideal for slow, uniform cooking, whereas stainless steel inserts are typically lighter and easier for transferring food to containers. Removable inserts make cleaning up after cooking easy, which is vital for keeping your kitchen clean. This guarantees that food preparation and cleanup are straightforward and efficient, making cooking for your dog as simple as possible.

Additionally, another factor to consider is the lid's design. A slow cooker with a secure locking lid is ideal for preventing spills, especially if you intend to travel with the cooker or keep the prepared food in the fridge. We prefer glass lids because they allow you to observe the cooking process without having to remove the lid and release heat. This feature aids in maintaining a consistent cooking temperature, guaranteeing that the food cooks correctly and uniformly.

Heat settings are another significant aspect. A suitable slow cooker should have at least three settings, including low, high, and keep warm. The low setting is ideal for slow-cooking tougher items such as root vegetables and meats, ensuring they become tender and delicious. When you don't have much time, utilize the high setting to cook faster dishes. The keep-warm setting keeps the food at a safe temperature until you're ready to feed it, which is very useful for preserving the nutritional value of the dog food.

When choosing a slow cooker, consider its safety features. Look for versions with cool-touch handles and non-slip feet to avoid kitchen accidents. An automated shut-off feature can provide an extra degree of safety, preventing the slow cooker from overheating if you forget to switch it off. These safety measures ensure that meal preparation is not only simple but also safe, giving you peace of mind as you prepare food for your pet.

Slow cookers have the practical advantage of being energy-efficient. These appliances use less electricity than standard ovens or stovetops, which can lower your utility expenses. For environmentally conscious pet owners, slow cookers, designed to cook food over long periods of time using low energy, are an environmentally beneficial option. This makes slow cooking a more sustainable option for making homemade dog food.

Incorporating a slow cooker into your routine makes it easier to prepare healthy, fresh meals for your dog. It combines simplicity, efficiency, and safety, allowing you to meet your pet's nutritional requirements without devoting your own time and energy. Using a slow cooker ensures your dog's health and happiness while also providing a practical, long-term option for your household. This deliberate approach to cooking ensures that your dog eats nutritious and delicious meals, promoting their health and well-being in the most efficient way possible.

Essential Tools and Equipment

When it comes to creating fresh meals for your dog, having the correct tools and equipment can help make the process go more smoothly and fun. Firstly, in addition to the slow cooker, a set of measuring cups and spoons is required to correctly distribute ingredients. Precise measures help to preserve the nutritional balance of the recipes, ensuring that your dog receives the appropriate amount of each component. Moreover, a digital kitchen scale may also be quite handy for weighing products such as meats and cereals, giving you confidence in the accuracy of your measurements.

Furthermore, a sharp knife and a solid cutting board are essential tools for preparing fresh food. Whether you're chopping vegetables or slicing meat, having high-quality tools may help you prepare food faster and more efficiently. Choose a non-slip cutting board for added safety while working.

Storage containers are another essential part of your cooking arsenal. After preparing a significant amount of food, you'll need a safe place to store it. BPA-free plastic containers or glass jars with tight-fitting lids are ideal for keeping food fresh in the fridge or freezer. Additionally, label each container with the date and contents to keep track of when each batch was prepared, ensuring that your dog always receives fresh food.

An immersion blender or food processor can be extremely useful for ensuring that the food has the proper consistency, particularly for elderly dogs or those with dental concerns. These tools let you purée or finely chop items, resulting in meals that are easier for your dog to consume and digest.

In addition, purchasing a high-quality ladle and serving spoon will make portioning food easier when it comes time to serve. A ladle with a spout can help reduce spillage, keeping your kitchen clean and meals more efficient.

A thermometer is useful for ensuring that food is prepared to the correct temperature, particularly when preparing meat. Keeping the inside temperature at a reasonable level is crucial for preventing foodborne infections. For those who enjoy multitasking, a set of silicone spatulas is ideal for stirring and scraping the sides of the slow cooker without harming the surface. These spatulas are heat-resistant and flexible, which renders them ideal for use with a slow cooker.

Finally, consider a recipe binder or diary. Keeping your favorite recipes, notes, and modifications separate simplifies cooking and lets you improve successful meals. This can also be a terrific way to share your favorite creations with other dog owners. Consequently, with the correct tools and equipment, preparing homemade dog food becomes a manageable and pleasurable practice. Each piece of equipment is essential for ensuring that your dog's meals are nutritional, safe, and enjoyable, improving their general health and enjoyment.

Preparing Ingredients for Slow Cooking

Cleaning and Preparing Vegetables

Preparing vegetables properly is an important step in ensuring that your dog's homemade meals are both nutritional and safe. Begin by sourcing fresh, high-quality veggies such as carrots, sweet potatoes, green beans, and spinach. These provide critical vitamins and minerals to help your dog's general wellness. Beforehand, properly wash them under running water to eliminate any dirt, pesticides, or pathogens. A vegetable brush can help ensure a more thorough cleaning, particularly for root vegetables such as carrots and potatoes.

Peeling some vegetables can be advantageous, but it isn't always essential. For example, you can peel sweet potatoes and carrots to remove dirt and enhance texture, but leaving the skin on preserves more nutrients and fiber. Additionally, if you wish to preserve the skin, make sure it is well cleaned to remove any residue. Afterwards, cut them into uniform pieces to ensure even cooking. This is especially crucial for slow cooking since it allows all components to cook at the same time, conserving nutritional content and increasing flavor.

Next, remove any rough stems from leafy greens such as spinach and kale, then slice the leaves into manageable pieces. These greens are rich in vitamins A, C, and K, which are essential for your dog's immune system and overall health. To preserve the beautiful color and nutritious value of these greens, add them near the end of the cooking process.

Using a sharp knife and a sturdy chopping board will make preparation easier and more fun. A sharp knife produces clean cuts and decreases the chance of harm, while a solid cutting board provides a safe work surface. Nonslip cutting boards are very beneficial since they remain in position while you chop.

Before adding some vegetables to the slow cooker, blanching them may be beneficial. Blanching involves briefly cooking vegetables and then immersing them in freezing water. This method helps to preserve their color, texture, and nutrients. For example, blanching green beans and broccoli might make them more appetizing and digestible for your dog.

Finally, you can add all the cleaned, peeled (if necessary), and chopped vegetables to the slow cooker. Layering ingredients carefully can help improve cooking results. Place denser vegetables like sweet potatoes and carrots at the bottom of the slow cooker to receive the most heat, and add more delicate veggies like spinach and green beans on top or near the end of the cooking time.

Preparing Meat

Preparing meat for slow cooking is essential for providing nutritious and appetizing meals for your dog. The process begins with the selection of high-quality meats such as chicken, beef, turkey, or lamb, which are abundant in proteins required for your dog's muscle development and overall wellness. Once you've decided on your meat, handling and preparing it correctly ensures safety and maximizes nutritional value.

If you have packaged and stored the meat for an extended period, it is crucial to thoroughly wash it in cold water to remove any impurities. To remove excess water from the meat, pat it dry with paper towels. This will help to produce better texture and flavor during slow cooking. Next, remove any visible fat, especially if your dog needs a low-fat diet. While a little fat is necessary for producing energy and maintaining a healthy coat, too much can cause digestive problems and obesity.

Using a sharp knife, carefully cut away any large bits of fat or gristle. This not only increases the meat's digestibility but also makes the meal more appealing to your dog. Cut the meat into uniform pieces about one to two inches in size. This ensures uniform and thorough cooking of the meat, which is crucial for both taste and safety. Smaller chunks make it easier for your dog to absorb and digest his food. Furthermore, marinating harder portions of meat in a dog-safe marinade, such as a mix of apple cider vinegar and water, will help tenderize and flavor the meat.

Before slow-cooking, brown the meat to boost its flavor and nutrients. Browning involves briefly cooking meat in a hot skillet with a little oil; sealing in fluids adds taste to the meal. Use small amounts of safe oils for dogs, such as coconut or olive oil. Moreover, before cooking the meat, remove any bones. Cooked bones can become brittle and splinter, providing a major choking threat and perhaps causing internal harm to your dog. Always use boneless cuts of meat; if you must use bone-in meat, make sure to remove the bones before serving.

In the meantime, strategically stack the meat with other ingredients in the slow cooker. Place denser vegetables like sweet potatoes and carrots at the bottom, followed by the meat, and then finish with lighter vegetables and greens. This stacking technique provides even cooking and maximum flavor dispersion.

Keeping a clean workspace is essential during the meat processing procedure. Use separate chopping boards and knives for meat and vegetables to avoid cross-contamination. Therefore, to preserve a sanitary cooking environment, make sure to wash your hands, any surfaces you touched, and any utensils you used after you've prepared the meat.

Portion Size for Nutritional Balance

Accurate portion sizes are vital for your dog's nutritional balance and wellness, helping to regulate weight and energy levels. The ideal portion varies by your dog's weight, age, and activity level, typically 2-3% of their body weight per day. For example, a 50-pound dog needs about one to one and a half pounds of food daily. Consult a veterinarian for precise recommendations.

Use both digital kitchen scales to accurately weigh meat and grains, as well as measuring cups and spoons, which are essential for portioning grains, vegetables, and oils. These tools allow you to follow recipes accurately while also maintaining the nutritional balance for precise portioning.

Consistent portion sizes support nutritional balance, simplify meal prep, and control costs. Moreover, preparing large batches in a slow cooker saves time and money, requiring precise ingredient measurement. This ensures that each batch has consistent nutritional content, making meal preparation efficient and helping with portion control when storing meals.

In addition, accurately measuring fat is critical. Using a tablespoon for oils like olive or coconut ensures you don't exceed the required amount, as excess fat can cause weight gain and digestive issues. Also, keeping a record of foods and quantities in each meal helps monitor your dog's weight, energy, and overall health, making it easier to adjust recipes while maintaining nutritional balance.

Cooking Time and Measurement Conversions

Making homemade meals for your dog involves precise measurement and cooking time to guarantee that each dish is successful. Precise measurement conversions are critical, especially if you're using a combination of metric and imperial measurements. For instance, recognizing that 1 cup equals approximately 240 milliliters helps with the consistency of liquid substances. Similarly, dry component measurements require converting 1 ounce to 28 grams.

Therefore, keeping a conversion chart on hand can be quite useful, especially when scaling recipes up or down to meet your dog's nutritional requirements. If a recipe calls for 500 grams of chicken, knowing that this amounts to around 1.1 pounds ensures that you use the exact amount while retaining the meal's desired nutritional balance.

Furthermore, correct measurement conversions aid in maintaining portion control, which is critical for dogs with special nutritional requirements or weight management concerns. For example, including the appropriate proportion of elements in a balanced meal, such as 50 grams of spinach (about 1.76 ounces), helps meet your dog's nutritional needs without overfeeding.

Adjusting cooking times is another important consideration, especially when using a slow cooker. The temperature and efficiency of slow cookers can vary, affecting how long it takes to fully cook dishes. As a general guideline, if a meal made on a high setting in one slow cooker takes 4 hours, it may take 6–8 hours on a low one. Always watch the first few batches to fine-tune cooking timings for your particular equipment. For example, if a Lamb and Lentil Soup recipe calls for 8 hours on low, check it at 6 hours to ensure even cooking and adjust the time as needed.

Moreover, certain foods may require cooking time alterations to maintain their nutritional value and texture. When you slightly undercook vegetables like carrots and sweet potatoes before freezing, they continue to cook during reheating, preserving their texture and nutrients. Incorporating these intricacies ensures that your dog's meals are both delicious and nutritious.

Chapter 4
Everyday Balanced Meals for Dogs

Chicken-Based Recipes

CHICKEN AND MANGO DELIGHT

INGREDIENTS

- 2 pounds of chicken (diced)
- 2 cups of mango (peeled and chopped)
- 1 cup of spinach (chopped)
- 1 cup of reduced quinoa (cooked)
- 1 teaspoon of ginger (finely grated)
- 2 cups of water

INSTRUCTIONS

1. Preparation:
Peel and chop the mango.
Chop the spinach.
Measure out the cooked quinoa.
Grate the ginger finely.

2. Layering Ingredients:
Place the diced chicken at the bottom of the slow cooker.
Add the mango, spinach, quinoa, and ginger on top of the chicken.
Pour in the water to ensure the ingredients are well-moistened.

3. Cooking:
Cover the slow cooker with the lid and set it to low heat.
Cook for 6-8 hours on low, or until the chicken is fully cooked and tender.

4. Final Touches:
Stir the mixture well to ensure even distribution of ingredients.
Allow to cool before serving.

PORTION CONTROL AND SIZE RECOMMENDATIONS:

Small Dogs: 1/2 cup per meal
Medium Dogs: 1 cup per meal
Large Dogs: 2 cups per meal

NUTRITIONAL INFORMATION AND CALORIE REQUIREMENTS:

Small Portion (1/2 cup):
Calories: 130 kcal
Protein: 18g
Fat: 4g
Carbohydrates: 8g

Medium Portion (1 cup):
Calories: 260 kcal
Protein: 36g
Fat: 8g
Carbohydrates: 16g

Large Portion (2 cups):
Calories: 520 kcal
Protein: 72g
Fat: 16g
Carbohydrates: 32g

ADAPTATIONS FOR DIFFERENT LIFE STAGES, BREEDS, AND ACTIVITY LEVELS:

Puppies:
Add an extra 1/2 cup of diced chicken to increase protein. Ensure the mixture is finely chopped for easier digestion.

Adults:
Follow the standard recipe.

Seniors:
Reduce protein slightly by removing 1/2 cup of chicken.
Add an extra 1/4 cup of quinoa for additional fiber.

High-Activity Dogs:
Increase portion size by 25% to meet higher energy needs.

Low-Activity Dogs:
Ensure portion control to prevent weight gain. Monitor and adjust based on the dog's activity and weight management needs.

CHICKEN AND BEET STEW

INGREDIENTS

- 2 pounds of chicken (diced)
- 2 cups of beets (peeled and chopped)
- 1 cup of green beans (chopped)
- 1 cup of cauliflower rice
- 1/2 teaspoon of turmeric
- 2 cups of water

INSTRUCTIONS

1. Preparation:
Peel and chop the beets.
Chop the green beans.
Measure out the cauliflower rice.

2. Layering Ingredients:
Place the diced chicken at the bottom of the slow cooker.
Add the beets, green beans, and cauliflower rice on top of the chicken.
Sprinkle the turmeric over the top.
Pour in the water to ensure the ingredients are well-moistened.

3. Cooking:
Cover the slow cooker with the lid and set it to low heat.
Cook for 6-8 hours on low, or until the chicken is fully cooked and tender.

4. Final Touches:
Stir the mixture well to ensure even distribution of ingredients.
Allow to cool before serving.

PORTION CONTROL AND SIZE RECOMMENDATIONS:

Small Dogs: 1/2 cup per meal
Medium Dogs: 1 cup per meal
Large Dogs: 2 cups per meal

NUTRITIONAL INFORMATION AND CALORIE REQUIREMENTS:

Small Portion (1/2 cup):
Calories: 135 kcal
Protein: 18g
Fat: 4g
Carbohydrates: 9g
Medium Portion (1 cup):
Calories: 270 kcal
Protein: 36g
Fat: 8g
Carbohydrates: 18g
Large Portion (2 cups):
Calories: 540 kcal
Protein: 72g
Fat: 16g
Carbohydrates: 36g

ADAPTATIONS FOR DIFFERENT LIFE STAGES, BREEDS, AND ACTIVITY LEVELS:

Puppies:
Add an extra 1/2 cup of diced chicken to increase protein.
Ensure the mixture is finely chopped for easier digestion.
Adults:
Follow the standard recipe.
Seniors:
Reduce protein slightly by removing 1/2 cup of chicken.
Add an extra 1/4 cup of cauliflower rice for additional fiber.
High-Activity Dogs:
Increase portion size by 25% to meet higher energy needs.
Low-Activity Dogs:
Ensure portion control to prevent weight gain.
Monitor and adjust based on the dog's activity and weight management needs.

CHICKEN AND SWEET POTATO DELIGHT

INGREDIENTS

- 2 pounds of chicken (diced)
- 2 cups of reduced sweet potatoes (peeled and cubed)
- 1 cup of peas (fresh or frozen)
- 2 tablespoons of parsley (chopped)
- 1/2 teaspoon of turmeric
- 2 cups of water

INSTRUCTIONS

1. Preparation:
Peel and cube the sweet potatoes.
Measure out the peas.
Chop the parsley.
2. Layering Ingredients:
Place the diced chicken at the bottom of the slow cooker.
Add the sweet potatoes, peas, and parsley on top of the chicken.
Sprinkle the turmeric over the top.
Pour in the water to ensure the ingredients are well-moistened.
3. Cooking:
Cover the slow cooker with the lid and set it to low heat.
Cook for 6-8 hours on low, or until the chicken is fully cooked and tender.
4. Touches:
Stir the mixture well to ensure even distribution of ingredients.
Allow to cool before serving.

PORTION CONTROL AND SIZE RECOMMENDATIONS:

Small Dogs: 1/2 cup per meal
Medium Dogs: 1 cup per meal
Large Dogs: 2 cups per meal

NUTRITIONAL INFORMATION AND CALORIE REQUIREMENTS:

Small Portion (1/2 cup):
Calories: 140 kcal
Protein: 18g
Fat: 4g
Carbohydrates: 10g
Medium Portion (1 cup):
Calories: 280 kcal
Protein: 36g
Fat: 8g
Carbohydrates: 20g
Large Portion (2 cups):
Calories: 560 kcal
Protein: 72g
Fat: 16g
Carbohydrates: 40g

ADAPTATIONS FOR DIFFERENT LIFE STAGES, BREEDS, AND ACTIVITY LEVELS:

Puppies:
Increase protein by adding an extra 1/2 cup of diced chicken.
Ensure the mixture is finely chopped for easier digestion.
Adults:
Follow the standard recipe.
Seniors:
Reduce the protein slightly by removing 1/2 cup of chicken.
Add an extra 1/4 cup of peas for additional fiber.
High-Activity Dogs:
Increase portion size by 25% to meet higher energy needs.
Low-Activity Dogs:
Ensure portion control to prevent weight gain.
Monitor and adjust based on the dog's activity and weight management needs.

HERBED CHICKEN AND ZUCCHINI

INGREDIENTS

- 2 pounds of chicken (diced)
- 1 cup of reduced quinoa (cooked)
- 1 teaspoon of rosemary (dried or fresh)
- 1 cup of zucchini (chopped)
- 1/2 teaspoon of basil
- 2 cups of water

INSTRUCTIONS

1. Preparation:
Dice the chicken.
Cook and measure the reduced quinoa.
Chop the zucchini.
Measure out the rosemary and basil.

2. Layering Ingredients:
Place the diced chicken at the bottom of the slow cooker.
Add the cooked quinoa and chopped zucchini on top of the chicken.
Sprinkle rosemary and basil over the mixture.
Pour in the water to ensure the ingredients are well-moistened.

3. Cooking:
Cover the slow cooker with the lid and set it to low heat.
Cook for 6-8 hours on low, or until the chicken is fully cooked and tender.

4. Final Touches:
Stir the mixture well to ensure even distribution of ingredients.
Allow to cool before serving.

PORTION CONTROL AND SIZE RECOMMENDATIONS:

Small Dogs: 1/2 cup per meal
Medium Dogs: 1 cup per meal
Large Dogs: 2 cups per meal

NUTRITIONAL INFORMATION AND CALORIE REQUIREMENTS:

Small Portion (1/2 cup):
Calories: 130 kcal
Protein: 18g
Fat: 4g
Carbohydrates: 8g
Medium Portion (1 cup):
Calories: 260 kcal
Protein: 36g
Fat: 8g
Carbohydrates: 16g
Large Portion (2 cups):
Calories: 520 kcal
Protein: 72g
Fat: 16g
Carbohydrates: 32g

ADAPTATIONS FOR DIFFERENT LIFE STAGES, BREEDS, AND ACTIVITY LEVELS:

Puppies:
Increase protein by adding an extra 1/2 cup of diced chicken.
Ensure the mixture is finely chopped for easier digestion.
Adults:
Follow the standard recipe.
Seniors:
Reduce the protein slightly by removing 1/2 cup of chicken.
Add an extra 1/4 cup of quinoa for additional fiber.
High-Activity Dogs:
Increase portion size by 25% to meet higher energy needs.
Low-Activity Dogs:
Ensure portion control to prevent weight gain.
Monitor and adjust based on the dog's activity and weight management needs.

CHICKEN AND BUTTERNUT SQUASH DELIGHT

INGREDIENTS 1 POUND OF CHICKEN (DICED)

1 cup of butternut squash (peeled and cubed)

1 cup of lentils (cooked)

1/2 cup of celery (chopped)

1 teaspoon of oregano

INSTRUCTIONS

1. Preparation:
Wash and chop all vegetables.
Rinse and cook the lentils according to package instructions if not already cooked.
2. Layering Ingredients: Place the diced chicken, cubed butternut squash, lentils and chopped celery into the slow cooker. Sprinkle the oregano over the mixture. Add enough water to cover the ingredients.
3. Cooking: Set the slow cooker to low heat. Cook for 6-8 hours or until the chicken is fully cooked and the vegetables are tender.
4. Final Touches:
Allow the mixture to cool completely before serving.
Store in an airtight container in the refrigerator.

PORTION CONTROL AND SIZE RECOMMENDATIONS: SMALL DOGS (10-20 LBS): 1/2 CUP PER MEAL

Medium Dogs (20-50 lbs): 1 cup per meal
Large Dogs (50+ lbs): 1 1/2 - 2 cups per meal

NUTRITIONAL INFORMATION AND CALORIE REQUIREMENTS:

Small Portion (1/2 cup):
Calories: 100 kcal
Protein: 10g
Fat: 2g
Carbohydrates: 12g
Medium Portion (1 cup):
Calories: 200 kcal
Protein: 20g
Fat: 4g
Carbohydrates: 24g
Large Portion (2 cups):
Calories: 400 kcal
Protein: 40g
Fat: 8g
Carbohydrates: 48g

ADAPTATIONS FOR DIFFERENT LIFE STAGES, BREEDS, AND ACTIVITY LEVELS:

Puppies:
Ensure the mixture is finely chopped for easier chewing and digestion. Consider increasing protein by adding an extra 1/4 cup of diced chicken.
Adults:
Follow the standard portion recommendations.
Seniors:
Reduce portion size by 25% to manage calorie intake.
Add an extra 1/4 cup of lentils for additional fiber.
High-Activity Dogs:
Increase portion size by 25% to meet higher energy needs.
Low-Activity Dogs: Reduce portion size by 25% to prevent overfeeding..

CHICKEN AND APPLE STEW

INGREDIENTS

- 2 pounds of chicken (diced)
- 2 cups of apples (chopped, seeds removed)
- 1 cup of carrots (chopped)
- 1/2 teaspoon of ginger (ground)
- 1/2 teaspoon of flaxseed (ground)
- 2 cups of water

INSTRUCTIONS

1. Preparation:
Dice the chicken.
Core and chop the apples.
Chop the carrots.
Measure out the ginger and flaxseed.

2. Layering Ingredients:
Place the diced chicken at the bottom of the slow cooker.
Add the apples and carrots on top of the chicken.
Sprinkle ginger and flaxseed over the mixture.
Pour in the water to ensure the ingredients are well-moistened.

3. Cooking:
Cover the slow cooker with the lid and set it to low heat.
Cook for 6-8 hours on low, or until the chicken is fully cooked and tender.

4. Final Touches:
Stir the mixture well to ensure even distribution of ingredients.
Allow to cool before serving.

PORTION CONTROL AND SIZE RECOMMENDATIONS:

Small Dogs: 1/2 cup per meal
Medium Dogs: 1 cup per meal
Large Dogs: 2 cups per meal

NUTRITIONAL INFORMATION AND CALORIE REQUIREMENTS:

Small Portion (1/2 cup):
Calories: 130 kcal
Protein: 18g
Fat: 4g
Carbohydrates: 10g
Medium Portion (1 cup):
Calories: 260 kcal
Protein: 36g
Fat: 8g
Carbohydrates: 20g
Large Portion (2 cups):
Calories: 520 kcal
Protein: 72g
Fat: 16g
Carbohydrates: 40g

ADAPTATIONS FOR DIFFERENT LIFE STAGES, BREEDS, AND ACTIVITY LEVELS:

Puppies:
Increase protein by adding an extra 1/2 cup of diced chicken.
Ensure the mixture is finely chopped for easier digestion.
Adults:
Follow the standard recipe.
Seniors:
Reduce protein slightly by removing 1/2 cup of chicken.
Add an extra 1/4 cup of carrots for additional fiber.
High-Activity Dogs:
Increase portion size by 25% to meet higher energy needs.
Low-Activity Dogs:
Ensure portion control to prevent weight gain.
Monitor and adjust based on the dog's activity and weight management needs.

CHICKEN AND KALE MIX

INGREDIENTS

- 2 pounds of chicken (diced)
- 1 cup of cauliflower rice
- 1 cup of kale (chopped)
- 1 cup of sweet corn (fresh or frozen)
- 2 tablespoons of parsley (chopped)
- 2 cups of water

INSTRUCTIONS

1. Preparation:
Dice the chicken.
Chop the kale and parsley.
Measure out the cauliflower rice and sweet corn.

2. Layering Ingredients:
Place the diced chicken at the bottom of the slow cooker.
Add the cauliflower rice, kale, sweet corn, and parsley on top.
Pour in the water to ensure the ingredients are well-moistened.

3. Cooking:
Cover the slow cooker with the lid and set it to low heat.
Cook for 6-8 hours on low, or until the chicken is fully cooked and tender.

4. Final Touches:
Stir the mixture well to ensure even distribution of ingredients.
Allow to cool before serving.

PORTION CONTROL AND SIZE RECOMMENDATIONS:

Small Dogs: 1/2 cup per meal
Medium Dogs: 1 cup per meal
Large Dogs: 2 cups per meal

NUTRITIONAL INFORMATION AND CALORIE REQUIREMENTS:

Small Portion (1/2 cup):
Calories: 130 kcal
Protein: 18g
Fat: 4g
Carbohydrates: 8g

Medium Portion (1 cup):
Calories: 260 kcal
Protein: 36g
Fat: 8g
Carbohydrates: 16g

Large Portion (2 cups):
Calories: 520 kcal
Protein: 72g
Fat: 16g
Carbohydrates: 32g

ADAPTATIONS FOR DIFFERENT LIFE STAGES, BREEDS, AND ACTIVITY LEVELS:

Puppies:
Increase protein by adding an extra 1/2 cup of diced chicken.
Ensure the mixture is finely chopped for easier digestion.

Adults:
Follow the standard recipe.

Seniors:
Reduce protein slightly by removing 1/2 cup of chicken.
Add an extra 1/4 cup of cauliflower rice for additional fiber.

High-Activity Dogs:
Increase portion size by 25% to meet higher energy needs.

Low-Activity Dogs:
Ensure portion control to prevent weight gain.
Monitor and adjust based on the dog's activity and weight management needs.

COCONUT CHICKEN AND VEGGIES

INGREDIENTS

- 2 pounds of chicken (diced)
- 1 cup of coconut milk (unsweetened)
- 1 cup of peas (fresh or frozen)
- 1 cup of carrots (chopped)
- 1/2 teaspoon of turmeric
- 2 cups of water

INSTRUCTIONS

1. Preparation:
Dice the chicken.
Chop the carrots.
Measure out the peas.

2. Layering Ingredients:
Place the diced chicken at the bottom of the slow cooker.
Add the peas and carrots on top of the chicken.
Sprinkle the turmeric over the top.
Pour in the coconut milk and water to ensure the ingredients are well-moistened.

3. Cooking:
Cover the slow cooker with the lid and set it to low heat.
Cook for 6-8 hours on low, or until the chicken is fully cooked and tender.

4. Final Touches:
Stir the mixture well to ensure even distribution of ingredients.
Allow to cool before serving.

PORTION CONTROL AND SIZE RECOMMENDATIONS:

Small Dogs: 1/2 cup per meal
Medium Dogs: 1 cup per meal
Large Dogs: 2 cups per meal

NUTRITIONAL INFORMATION AND CALORIE REQUIREMENTS:

Small Portion (1/2 cup):
Calories: 140 kcal
Protein: 19g
Fat: 5g
Carbohydrates: 8g
Medium Portion (1 cup):
Calories: 280 kcal
Protein: 38g
Fat: 10g
Carbohydrates: 16g
Large Portion (2 cups):
Calories: 560 kcal
Protein: 76g
Fat: 20g
Carbohydrates: 32g

ADAPTATIONS FOR DIFFERENT LIFE STAGES, BREEDS, AND ACTIVITY LEVELS:

Puppies:
Increase protein by adding an extra 1/2 cup of diced chicken.
Ensure the mixture is finely chopped for easier digestion.
Adults:
Follow the standard recipe.
Seniors:
Reduce protein slightly by removing 1/2 cup of chicken.
Add an extra 1/4 cup of peas for additional fiber.
High-Activity Dogs:
Increase portion size by 25% to meet higher energy needs.
Low-Activity Dogs:
Ensure portion control to prevent weight gain.
Monitor and adjust based on the dog's activity and weight management needs.

CHICKEN AND CHICKPEA COMBO

INGREDIENTS

- 2 pounds of chicken (diced)
- 1 cup of reduced chickpeas (cooked)
- 1 cup of spinach (chopped)
- 2 tablespoons of parsley (chopped)
- 1/2 teaspoon of cumin
- 2 cups of water

INSTRUCTIONS

1. Preparation:
Dice the chicken.
Chop the spinach and parsley.
Measure out the cooked chickpeas.

2. Layering Ingredients:
Place the diced chicken at the bottom of the slow cooker.
Add the chickpeas, spinach, and parsley on top of the chicken.
Sprinkle the cumin over the top.
Pour in the water to ensure the ingredients are well-moistened.

3. Cooking:
Cover the slow cooker with the lid and set it to low heat.
Cook for 6-8 hours on low, or until the chicken is fully cooked and tender.

4. Final Touches:
Stir the mixture well to ensure even distribution of ingredients.
Allow to cool before serving.

PORTION CONTROL AND SIZE RECOMMENDATIONS:

Small Dogs: 1/2 cup per meal
Medium Dogs: 1 cup per meal
Large Dogs: 2 cups per meal

NUTRITIONAL INFORMATION AND CALORIE REQUIREMENTS:

Small Portion (1/2 cup):
Calories: 145 kcal
Protein: 18g
Fat: 5g
Carbohydrates: 9g

Medium Portion (1 cup):
Calories: 290 kcal
Protein: 36g
Fat: 10g
Carbohydrates: 18g

Large Portion (2 cups):
Calories: 580 kcal
Protein: 72g
Fat: 20g
Carbohydrates: 36g

ADAPTATIONS FOR DIFFERENT LIFE STAGES, BREEDS, AND ACTIVITY LEVELS:

Puppies:
Increase protein by adding an extra 1/2 cup of diced chicken.
Ensure the mixture is finely chopped for easier digestion.

Adults:
Follow the standard recipe.

Seniors:
Reduce protein slightly by removing 1/2 cup of chicken.
Add an extra 1/4 cup of chickpeas for additional fiber.

High-Activity Dogs:
Increase portion size by 25% to meet higher energy needs.

Low-Activity Dogs:
Ensure portion control to prevent weight gain.
Monitor and adjust based on the dog's activity and weight management needs.

CHICKEN AND SPINACH DELIGHT

INGREDIENTS

- 2 pounds of chicken (diced)
- 1 cup of cauliflower rice
- 1 cup of carrots (chopped)
- 1 cup of spinach (chopped)
- 1/2 teaspoon of thyme
- 2 cups of water

INSTRUCTIONS

1. Preparation:
Dice the chicken.
Chop the carrots and spinach.
Measure out the cauliflower rice.

2. Layering Ingredients:
Place the diced chicken at the bottom of the slow cooker.
Add the cauliflower rice, carrots, and spinach on top of the chicken.
Sprinkle the thyme over the top.
Pour in the water to ensure the ingredients are well-moistened.

3. Cooking:
Cover the slow cooker with the lid and set it to low heat.
Cook for 6-8 hours on low, or until the chicken is fully cooked and tender.

4. Final Touches:
Stir the mixture well to ensure even distribution of ingredients.
Allow to cool before serving.

PORTION CONTROL AND SIZE RECOMMENDATIONS:

Small Dogs: 1/2 cup per meal
Medium Dogs: 1 cup per meal
Large Dogs: 2 cups per meal

NUTRITIONAL INFORMATION AND CALORIE REQUIREMENTS:

Small Portion (1/2 cup):
Calories: 130 kcal
Protein: 18g
Fat: 4g
Carbohydrates: 8g

Medium Portion (1 cup):
Calories: 260 kcal
Protein: 36g
Fat: 8g
Carbohydrates: 16g

Large Portion (2 cups):
Calories: 520 kcal
Protein: 72g
Fat: 16g
Carbohydrates: 32g

ADAPTATIONS FOR DIFFERENT LIFE STAGES, BREEDS, AND ACTIVITY LEVELS:

Puppies:
Increase protein by adding an extra 1/2 cup of diced chicken.
Ensure the mixture is finely chopped for easier digestion.

Adults:
Follow the standard recipe.

Seniors:
Reduce protein slightly by removing 1/2 cup of chicken.
Add an extra 1/4 cup of cauliflower rice for additional fiber.

High-Activity Dogs:
Increase portion size by 25% to meet higher energy needs.

Low-Activity Dogs:
Ensure portion control to prevent weight gain.
Monitor and adjust based on the dog's activity and weight management needs.

TURKEY AND BUTTERNUT SQUASH MIX

INGREDIENTS

- 2 pounds of turkey (diced)
- 1 cup of sweet corn
- 1 cup of butternut squash (peeled and cubed)
- 1 cup of spinach (chopped)
- 1/2 teaspoon of turmeric
- 2 cups of water

INSTRUCTIONS

1. Preparation:
Dice the turkey.
Peel and cube the butternut squash.
Chop the spinach.

2. Layering Ingredients:
Place the diced turkey at the bottom of the slow cooker.
Add the sweet corn, butternut squash, and spinach on top of the turkey.
Sprinkle the turmeric over the top.
Pour in the water to ensure the ingredients are well-moistened.

3. Cooking:
Cover the slow cooker with the lid and set it to low heat.
Cook for 6-8 hours on low, or until the turkey is fully cooked and tender.

4. Final Touches:
Stir the mixture well to ensure even distribution of ingredients.
Allow to cool before serving.

PORTION CONTROL AND SIZE RECOMMENDATIONS:

Small Dogs: 1/2 cup per meal
Medium Dogs: 1 cup per meal
Large Dogs: 2 cups per meal

NUTRITIONAL INFORMATION AND CALORIE REQUIREMENTS:

Small Portion (1/2 cup):
Calories: 135 kcal
Protein: 16g
Fat: 3g
Carbohydrates: 10g

Medium Portion (1 cup):
Calories: 270 kcal
Protein: 32g
Fat: 6g
Carbohydrates: 20g

Large Portion (2 cups):
Calories: 540 kcal
Protein: 64g
Fat: 12g
Carbohydrates: 40g

ADAPTATIONS FOR DIFFERENT LIFE STAGES, BREEDS, AND ACTIVITY LEVELS:

Puppies:
Increase protein by adding an extra 1/2 cup of diced turkey.
Ensure the mixture is finely chopped for easier digestion.

Adults:
Follow the standard recipe.

Seniors:
Reduce protein slightly by removing 1/2 cup of turkey.
Add an extra 1/4 cup of butternut squash for additional fiber.

High-Activity Dogs:
Increase portion size by 25% to meet higher energy needs.

Low-Activity Dogs:
Ensure portion control to prevent weight gain.
Monitor and adjust based on the dog's activity and weight management needs.

HERB-INFUSED TURKEY STEW

INGREDIENTS

- 2 pounds of turkey (diced)
- 1 cup of carrots (chopped)
- 1 cup of reduced lentils (cooked)
- 1 teaspoon of rosemary
- 1/2 teaspoon of thyme
- 2 cups of water

INSTRUCTIONS

1. Preparation:
Dice the turkey.
Chop the carrots.
Measure out the cooked lentils.

2. Layering Ingredients:
Place the diced turkey at the bottom of the slow cooker.
Add the carrots and lentils on top of the turkey.
Sprinkle the rosemary and thyme over the top.
Pour in the water to ensure the ingredients are well-moistened.

3. Cooking:
Cover the slow cooker with the lid and set it to low heat.
Cook for 6-8 hours on low, or until the turkey is fully cooked and tender.

4. Final Touches:
Stir the mixture well to ensure even distribution of ingredients.
Allow to cool before serving.

PORTION CONTROL AND SIZE RECOMMENDATIONS:

Small Dogs: 1/2 cup per meal
Medium Dogs: 1 cup per meal
Large Dogs: 2 cups per meal

NUTRITIONAL INFORMATION AND CALORIE REQUIREMENTS:

Small Portion (1/2 cup):
Calories: 140 kcal
Protein: 18g
Fat: 4g
Carbohydrates: 10g

Medium Portion (1 cup):
Calories: 280 kcal
Protein: 36g
Fat: 8g
Carbohydrates: 20g

Large Portion (2 cups):
Calories: 560 kcal
Protein: 72g
Fat: 16g
Carbohydrates: 40g

ADAPTATIONS FOR DIFFERENT LIFE STAGES, BREEDS, AND ACTIVITY LEVELS:

Puppies:
Increase protein by adding an extra 1/2 cup of diced turkey.
Ensure the mixture is finely chopped for easier digestion.

Adults:
Follow the standard recipe.

Seniors:
Reduce protein slightly by removing 1/2 cup of turkey.
Add an extra 1/4 cup of carrots for additional fiber.

High-Activity Dogs:
Increase portion size by 25% to meet higher energy needs.

Low-Activity Dogs:
Ensure portion control to prevent weight gain.
Monitor and adjust based on the dog's activity and weight management needs.

TURKEY AND PUMPKIN STEW

INGREDIENTS

- 2 pounds of turkey (diced)
- 1 cup of pumpkin (cooked and mashed)
- 1 cup of apples (cored and chopped)
- 1 cup of kale (chopped)
- 1/2 teaspoon of ginger (ground)
- 2 cups of water

INSTRUCTIONS

1. Preparation:
Dice the turkey.
Cook and mash the pumpkin.
Core and chop the apples.
Chop the kale.

2. Layering Ingredients:
Place the diced turkey at the bottom of the slow cooker.
Add the mashed pumpkin, chopped apples, and kale on top of the turkey.
Sprinkle the ginger evenly over the mixture.
Pour in the water to ensure the ingredients are well-moistened.

3. Cooking:
Cover the slow cooker with the lid and set it to low heat.
Cook for 6-8 hours on low, or until the turkey is fully cooked and tender.

4. Final Touches:
Stir the mixture well to ensure even distribution of ingredients.
Allow to cool before serving.

PORTION CONTROL AND SIZE RECOMMENDATIONS:

Small Dogs: 1/2 cup per meal
Medium Dogs: 1 cup per meal
Large Dogs: 2 cups per meal

NUTRITIONAL INFORMATION AND CALORIE REQUIREMENTS:

Small Portion (1/2 cup):
Calories: 120 kcal
Protein: 15g
Fat: 4g
Carbohydrates: 6g

Medium Portion (1 cup):
Calories: 240 kcal
Protein: 30g
Fat: 8g
Carbohydrates: 12g

Large Portion (2 cups):
Calories: 480 kcal
Protein: 60g
Fat: 16g
Carbohydrates: 24g

ADAPTATIONS FOR DIFFERENT LIFE STAGES, BREEDS, AND ACTIVITY LEVELS:

Puppies:
Increase protein by adding an extra 1/4 cup of diced turkey.
Ensure the mixture is finely chopped for easier digestion.

Adults:
Follow the standard recipe.

Seniors:
Reduce protein slightly by removing 1/4 cup of turkey.
Add an extra 1/4 cup of pumpkin for additional fiber.

High-Activity Dogs:
Increase portion size by 25% to meet higher energy needs.

Low-Activity Dogs:
Ensure portion control to prevent weight gain.
Monitor and adjust based on the dog's activity and weight management needs.

TURKEY AND CRANBERRY MIX

INGREDIENTS

- 2 pounds of turkey (diced)
- 1 cup of cranberries (fresh or frozen)
- 1 cup of reduced sweet potatoes (cooked and mashed)
- 1 cup of spinach (chopped)
- 1 teaspoon of ginger (finely grated)
- 2 cups of water

INSTRUCTIONS

1. Preparation:
Dice the turkey.
Cook and mash the sweet potatoes.
Chop the spinach.
Grate the ginger.

2. Layering Ingredients:
Place the diced turkey at the bottom of the slow cooker.
Add the cranberries, mashed sweet potatoes, and chopped spinach on top of the turkey.
Sprinkle the grated ginger over the mixture.
Pour in the water to ensure the ingredients are well-moistened.

3. Cooking:
Cover the slow cooker with the lid and set it to low heat.
Cook for 6-8 hours on low, or until the turkey is fully cooked and tender.

4. Final Touches:
Stir the mixture well to ensure even distribution of ingredients.
Allow to cool before serving.

PORTION CONTROL AND SIZE RECOMMENDATIONS:

Small Dogs: 1/2 cup per meal
Medium Dogs: 1 cup per meal
Large Dogs: 2 cups per meal

NUTRITIONAL INFORMATION AND CALORIE REQUIREMENTS:

Small Portion (1/2 cup):
Calories: 130 kcal
Protein: 14g
Fat: 4g
Carbohydrates: 10g

Medium Portion (1 cup):
Calories: 260 kcal
Protein: 28g
Fat: 8g
Carbohydrates: 20g

Large Portion (2 cups):
Calories: 520 kcal
Protein: 56g
Fat: 16g
Carbohydrates: 40g

ADAPTATIONS FOR DIFFERENT LIFE STAGES, BREEDS, AND ACTIVITY LEVELS:

Puppies:
Increase protein by adding an extra 1/4 cup of diced turkey.
Ensure the mixture is finely chopped for easier digestion.

Adults:
Follow the standard recipe.

Seniors:
Reduce protein slightly by removing 1/4 cup of turkey.
Add an extra 1/4 cup of sweet potatoes for additional fiber.

High-Activity Dogs:
Increase portion size by 25% to meet higher energy needs.

Low-Activity Dogs:
Ensure portion control to prevent weight gain.
Monitor and adjust based on the dog's activity and weight management needs.

TURKEY AND SPINACH DELIGHT

INGREDIENTS

- 2 pounds of turkey (diced)
- 1 cup of cauliflower rice
- 1 cup of peas (fresh or frozen)
- 1 cup of carrots (chopped)
- 1/2 teaspoon of basil
- 2 cups of water

INSTRUCTIONS

1. Preparation:
Dice the turkey.
Prepare the cauliflower rice.
Chop the carrots.
Measure out the peas.

2. Layering Ingredients:
Place the diced turkey at the bottom of the slow cooker.
Add the cauliflower rice, peas, and chopped carrots on top of the turkey.
Sprinkle the basil evenly over the mixture.
Pour in the water to ensure the ingredients are well-moistened.

3. Cooking:
Cover the slow cooker with the lid and set it to low heat.
Cook for 6-8 hours on low, or until the turkey is fully cooked and tender.

4. Final Touches:
Stir the mixture well to ensure even distribution of ingredients.
Allow to cool before serving.

PORTION CONTROL AND SIZE RECOMMENDATIONS:

Small Dogs: 1/2 cup per meal
Medium Dogs: 1 cup per meal
Large Dogs: 2 cups per meal

NUTRITIONAL INFORMATION AND CALORIE REQUIREMENTS:

Small Portion (1/2 cup):
Calories: 110 kcal
Protein: 14g
Fat: 3g
Carbohydrates: 6g

Medium Portion (1 cup):
Calories: 220 kcal
Protein: 28g
Fat: 6g
Carbohydrates: 12g

Large Portion (2 cups):
Calories: 440 kcal
Protein: 56g
Fat: 12g
Carbohydrates: 24g

ADAPTATIONS FOR DIFFERENT LIFE STAGES, BREEDS, AND ACTIVITY LEVELS:

Puppies:
Increase protein by adding an extra 1/4 cup of diced turkey.
Ensure the mixture is finely chopped for easier digestion.

Adults:
Follow the standard recipe.

Seniors:
Reduce protein slightly by removing 1/4 cup of turkey.
Add an extra 1/4 cup of peas for additional fiber.

High-Activity Dogs:
Increase portion size by 25% to meet higher energy needs.

Low-Activity Dogs:
Ensure portion control to prevent weight gain.
Monitor and adjust based on the dog's activity and weight management needs.

TURKEY AND PEAR DELIGHT

INGREDIENTS

- 2 pounds of turkey (ground)
- 2 ripe pears (cored and chopped)
- 1 cup of green beans (chopped)
- 1/2 cup of quinoa (rinsed and reduced)
- 1 tablespoon of fresh parsley (chopped)

INSTRUCTIONS

1. Preparation:
Wash and chop all vegetables and fruits.
Rinse and reduce the quinoa as per package instructions.

2. Layering Ingredients:
Place the ground turkey at the bottom of the slow cooker.
Add the chopped pears, green beans, and quinoa.
Sprinkle the chopped parsley on top.

3. Cooking:
Set the slow cooker to low heat and cook for 6-8 hours or until the turkey is fully cooked and the quinoa is tender.
Stir occasionally, if possible.

4. Final Touches:
Stir the mixture well to ensure even distribution of ingredients.
Allow to cool before serving.

PORTION CONTROL AND SIZE RECOMMENDATIONS:

Small Dogs (10-20 lbs): 1/2 cup per meal
Medium Dogs (20-50 lbs): 1 cup per meal
Large Dogs (50+ lbs): 1 1/2 - 2 cups per meal

NUTRITIONAL INFORMATION AND CALORIE REQUIREMENTS:

Small Portion (1/2 cup):
Calories: 150 kcal
Protein: 12g
Fat: 7g
Carbohydrates: 8g

Medium Portion (1 cup):
Calories: 300 kcal
Protein: 24g
Fat: 14g
Carbohydrates: 16g

Large Portion (2 cups):
Calories: 600 kcal
Protein: 48g
Fat: 28g
Carbohydrates: 32g

ADAPTATIONS FOR DIFFERENT LIFE STAGES, BREEDS, AND ACTIVITY LEVELS:

Puppies:
Increase protein by adding an extra 1/4 cup of ground turkey.
Ensure the mixture is finely chopped for easier digestion.

Adults:
Follow the standard recipe.

Seniors:
Reduce protein slightly by removing 1/4 cup of turkey.
Add an extra 1/4 cup of chopped green beans for additional fiber.

High-Activity Dogs:
Increase portion size by 25% to meet higher energy needs.

Low-Activity Dogs:
Reduce portion size by 25% to prevent overfeeding.

TURKEY AND CHICKPEA CASSEROLE

INGREDIENTS

- 2 pounds of turkey (ground)
- 1 cup of chickpeas (cooked and reduced)
- 1 cup of spinach (chopped)
- 1 tablespoon of fresh parsley (chopped)
- 1/2 teaspoon of cumin

INSTRUCTIONS

1. Preparation:
Wash and chop all vegetables.
Cook and reduce the chickpeas as per package instructions.

2. Layering Ingredients:
Place the ground turkey at the bottom of the slow cooker.
Add the reduced chickpeas and chopped spinach.
Sprinkle the chopped parsley and cumin on top.

3. Cooking:
Set the slow cooker to low heat and cook for 6-8 hours or until the turkey is fully cooked and the chickpeas are tender.
Stir occasionally if possible.

4. Final Touches:
Stir the mixture well to ensure even distribution of ingredients.
Allow to cool before serving.

PORTION CONTROL AND SIZE RECOMMENDATIONS:

Small Dogs (10-20 lbs): 1/2 cup per meal
Medium Dogs (20-50 lbs): 1 cup per meal
Large Dogs (50+ lbs): 1 1/2 - 2 cups per meal

NUTRITIONAL INFORMATION AND CALORIE REQUIREMENTS:

Small Portion (1/2 cup):
Calories: 160 kcal
Protein: 14g
Fat: 6g
Carbohydrates: 10g

Medium Portion (1 cup):
Calories: 320 kcal
Protein: 28g
Fat: 12g
Carbohydrates: 20g

Large Portion (2 cups):
Calories: 640 kcal
Protein: 56g
Fat: 24g
Carbohydrates: 40g

ADAPTATIONS FOR DIFFERENT LIFE STAGES, BREEDS, AND ACTIVITY LEVELS:

Puppies:
Increase protein by adding an extra 1/4 cup of ground turkey.
Ensure the mixture is finely chopped for easier digestion.

Adults:
Follow the standard recipe.

Seniors:
Reduce protein slightly by removing 1/4 cup of turkey.
Add an extra 1/4 cup of chopped spinach for additional fiber.

High-Activity Dogs:
Increase portion size by 25% to meet higher energy needs.

Low-Activity Dogs:
Reduce portion size by 25% to prevent overfeeding.

CITRUS TURKEY AND VEGGIES

INGREDIENTS

- 2 pounds of turkey (ground)
- 2 oranges (peeled and chopped)
- 1 cup of green beans (chopped)
- 1 cup of cauliflower rice
- 1 teaspoon of dill

INSTRUCTIONS

1. Preparation:
Wash and chop all vegetables and fruits.
Prepare the cauliflower rice as per package instructions.

2. Layering Ingredients:
Place the ground turkey at the bottom of the slow cooker.
Add the chopped oranges, green beans, and cauliflower rice.
Sprinkle the dill on top.

3. Cooking:
Set the slow cooker to low heat and cook for 6-8 hours or until the turkey is fully cooked and the vegetables are tender.
Stir occasionally if possible.

4. Final Touches:
Stir the mixture well to ensure even distribution of ingredients.
Allow to cool before serving.

PORTION CONTROL AND SIZE RECOMMENDATIONS:

Small Dogs (10-20 lbs): 1/2 cup per meal
Medium Dogs (20-50 lbs): 1 cup per meal
Large Dogs (50+ lbs): 1 1/2 - 2 cups per meal

NUTRITIONAL INFORMATION AND CALORIE REQUIREMENTS:

Small Portion (1/2 cup):
Calories: 145 kcal
Protein: 12g
Fat: 6g
Carbohydrates: 9g

Medium Portion (1 cup):
Calories: 290 kcal
Protein: 24g
Fat: 12g
Carbohydrates: 18g

Large Portion (2 cups):
Calories: 580 kcal
Protein: 48g
Fat: 24g
Carbohydrates: 36g

ADAPTATIONS FOR DIFFERENT LIFE STAGES, BREEDS, AND ACTIVITY LEVELS:

Puppies:
Increase protein by adding an extra 1/4 cup of ground turkey.
Ensure the mixture is finely chopped for easier digestion.

Adults:
Follow the standard recipe.

Seniors:
Reduce protein slightly by removing 1/4 cup of turkey.
Add an extra 1/4 cup of chopped green beans for additional fiber.

High-Activity Dogs:
Increase portion size by 25% to meet higher energy needs.

Low-Activity Dogs:
Reduce portion size by 25% to prevent overfeeding.

SAVORY TURKEY AND ZUCCHINI

INGREDIENTS

- 2 pounds of turkey (ground)
- 1 cup of reduced barley
- 1 cup of celery (chopped)
- 1 cup of zucchini (chopped)
- 1/2 teaspoon of rosemary

INSTRUCTIONS

1. Preparation:
Wash and chop all vegetables.
Rinse and reduce the barley as per package instructions.

2. Layering Ingredients:
Place the ground turkey at the bottom of the slow cooker.
Add the reduced barley, chopped celery, and zucchini.
Sprinkle the rosemary on top.

3. Cooking:
Cover the slow cooker with the lid.
Set the slow cooker to low heat and cook for 6-8 hours or until the turkey is fully cooked and the barley is tender.

4. Final Touches:
Stir the mixture well to ensure even distribution of ingredients.
Allow to cool before serving.

PORTION CONTROL AND SIZE RECOMMENDATIONS:

Small Dogs (10-20 lbs): 1/2 cup per meal
Medium Dogs (20-50 lbs): 1 cup per meal
Large Dogs (50+ lbs): 1 1/2 - 2 cups per meal

NUTRITIONAL INFORMATION AND CALORIE REQUIREMENTS:

Small Portion (1/2 cup):
Calories: 150 kcal
Protein: 13g
Fat: 6g
Carbohydrates: 10g
Medium Portion (1 cup):
Calories: 300 kcal
Protein: 26g
Fat: 12g
Carbohydrates: 20g
Large Portion (2 cups):
Calories: 600 kcal
Protein: 52g
Fat: 24g
Carbohydrates: 40g

ADAPTATIONS FOR DIFFERENT LIFE STAGES, BREEDS, AND ACTIVITY LEVELS:

Puppies:
Increase protein by adding an extra 1/4 cup of ground turkey.
Ensure the mixture is finely chopped for easier digestion.
Adults:
Follow the standard recipe.
Seniors:
Reduce protein slightly by removing 1/4 cup of turkey.
Add an extra 1/4 cup of chopped zucchini for additional fiber.
High-Activity Dogs:
Increase portion size by 25% to meet higher energy needs.
Low-Activity Dogs:
Reduce portion size by 25% to prevent overfeeding.

TURKEY AND PARSNIP BLEND

INGREDIENTS

- 2 pounds of turkey (ground)
- 1 cup of parsnips (chopped)
- 1 cup of carrots (chopped)
- 1/2 cup of reduced quinoa
- 1/2 teaspoon of oregano

INSTRUCTIONS

1. Preparation:
Wash and chop all vegetables.
Rinse and reduce the quinoa as per package instructions.

2. Layering Ingredients:
Place the ground turkey at the bottom of the slow cooker.
Add the chopped parsnips, carrots, and reduced quinoa.
Sprinkle the oregano on top.

3. Cooking:
Cover the slow cooker with the lid.
Set the slow cooker to low heat and cook for 6-8 hours or until the turkey is fully cooked and the vegetables are tender.

4. Final Touches:
Stir the mixture well to ensure even distribution of ingredients.
Allow to cool before serving.

PORTION CONTROL AND SIZE RECOMMENDATIONS:

Small Dogs (10-20 lbs): 1/2 cup per meal
Medium Dogs (20-50 lbs): 1 cup per meal
Large Dogs (50+ lbs): 1 1/2 - 2 cups per meal

NUTRITIONAL INFORMATION AND CALORIE REQUIREMENTS:

Small Portion (1/2 cup):
Calories: 160 kcal
Protein: 14g
Fat: 7g
Carbohydrates: 9g

Medium Portion (1 cup):
Calories: 320 kcal
Protein: 28g
Fat: 14g
Carbohydrates: 18g

Large Portion (2 cups):
Calories: 640 kcal
Protein: 56g
Fat: 28g
Carbohydrates: 36g

ADAPTATIONS FOR DIFFERENT LIFE STAGES, BREEDS, AND ACTIVITY LEVELS:

Puppies:
Increase protein by adding an extra 1/4 cup of ground turkey.
Ensure the mixture is finely chopped for easier digestion.

Adults:
Follow the standard recipe.

Seniors:
Reduce protein slightly by removing 1/4 cup of turkey.
Add an extra 1/4 cup of chopped carrots for additional fiber.

High-Activity Dogs:
Increase portion size by 25% to meet higher energy needs.

Low-Activity Dogs:
Reduce portion size by 25% to prevent overfeeding.

BEEF AND SWEET POTATO DELIGHT

INGREDIENTS

- 2 pounds of beef (ground or diced)
- 1 cup of reduced sweet potatoes (peeled and cubed)
- 1 cup of carrots (chopped)
- 1 cup of reduced quinoa (cooked)
- 1/2 teaspoon of oregano
- 1/2 teaspoon of basil
- 2 cups of water

INSTRUCTIONS

1. Preparation:
Dice or ground the beef.
Peel and cube the sweet potatoes.
Chop the carrots.
Measure out the cooked quinoa.

2. Layering Ingredients:
Place the beef at the bottom of the slow cooker.
Add the sweet potatoes, carrots, and quinoa on top of the beef.
Sprinkle the oregano and basil over the top.
Pour in the water to ensure the ingredients are well-moistened.

3. Cooking:
Cover the slow cooker with the lid and set it to low heat.
Cook for 6-8 hours on low, or until the beef is fully cooked and tender.

4. Final Touches:
Stir the mixture well to ensure even distribution of ingredients.
Allow to cool before serving.

PORTION CONTROL AND SIZE RECOMMENDATIONS:

Small Dogs: 1/2 cup per meal
Medium Dogs: 1 cup per meal
Large Dogs: 2 cups per meal

NUTRITIONAL INFORMATION AND CALORIE REQUIREMENTS:

Small Portion (1/2 cup):
Calories: 150 kcal
Protein: 21g
Fat: 5g
Carbohydrates: 10g

Medium Portion (1 cup):
Calories: 300 kcal
Protein: 42g
Fat: 10g
Carbohydrates: 20g

Large Portion (2 cups):
Calories: 600 kcal
Protein: 84g
Fat: 20g
Carbohydrates: 40g

ADAPTATIONS FOR DIFFERENT LIFE STAGES, BREEDS, AND ACTIVITY LEVELS:

Puppies:
Increase protein by adding an extra 1/2 cup of diced beef.
Ensure the mixture is finely chopped for easier digestion.

Adults:
Follow the standard recipe.

Seniors:
Reduce protein slightly by removing 1/2 cup of beef.
Add an extra 1/4 cup of sweet potatoes for additional fiber.

High-Activity Dogs:
Increase portion size by 25% to meet higher energy needs.

Low-Activity Dogs:
Ensure portion control to prevent weight gain.
Monitor and adjust based on the dog's activity and weight management needs.

BEEF AND LENTIL MIX

INGREDIENTS

- 2 pounds of beef (ground or diced)
- 1 cup of reduced lentils (cooked)
- 1 cup of green beans (chopped)
- 2 tablespoons of parsley (chopped)
- 1/2 teaspoon of turmeric
- 2 cups of water

INSTRUCTIONS

1. Preparation:
Dice or ground the beef.
Chop the green beans.
Measure out the cooked lentils.

2. Layering Ingredients:
Place the beef at the bottom of the slow cooker.
Add the lentils, green beans, and parsley on top of the beef.
Sprinkle the turmeric over the top.
Pour in the water to ensure the ingredients are well-moistened.

3. Cooking:
Cover the slow cooker with the lid and set it to low heat.
Cook for 6-8 hours on low, or until the beef is fully cooked and tender.

4. Final Touches:
Stir the mixture well to ensure even distribution of ingredients.
Allow to cool before serving.

PORTION CONTROL AND SIZE RECOMMENDATIONS:

Small Dogs: 1/2 cup per meal
Medium Dogs: 1 cup per meal
Large Dogs: 2 cups per meal

NUTRITIONAL INFORMATION AND CALORIE REQUIREMENTS:

Small Portion (1/2 cup):
Calories: 145 kcal
Protein: 20g
Fat: 5g
Carbohydrates: 8g

Medium Portion (1 cup):
Calories: 290 kcal
Protein: 40g
Fat: 10g
Carbohydrates: 16g

Large Portion (2 cups):
Calories: 580 kcal
Protein: 80g
Fat: 20g
Carbohydrates: 32g

ADAPTATIONS FOR DIFFERENT LIFE STAGES, BREEDS, AND ACTIVITY LEVELS:

Puppies:
Increase protein by adding an extra 1/2 cup of diced beef.
Ensure the mixture is finely chopped for easier digestion.

Adults:
Follow the standard recipe.

Seniors:
Reduce protein slightly by removing 1/2 cup of beef.
Add an extra 1/4 cup of lentils for additional fiber.

High-Activity Dogs:
Increase portion size by 25% to meet higher energy needs.

Low-Activity Dogs:
Ensure portion control to prevent weight gain.
Monitor and adjust based on the dog's activity and weight management needs.

BEEF AND BUTTERNUT SQUASH STEW

INGREDIENTS

- 2 pounds of beef (ground or diced)
- 1 cup of butternut squash (peeled and cubed)
- 1/2 cup of blueberries
- 1 cup of kale (chopped)
- 1/2 teaspoon of ginger (ground)
- 2 cups of water

INSTRUCTIONS

1. Preparation:
Dice or ground the beef.
Peel and cube the butternut squash.
Measure out the blueberries.
Chop the kale.

2. Layering Ingredients:
Place the beef at the bottom of the slow cooker.
Add the butternut squash, blueberries, and kale on top of the beef.
Sprinkle the ginger over the top.
Pour in the water to ensure the ingredients are well-moistened.

3. Cooking:
Cover the slow cooker with the lid and set it to low heat.
Cook for 6-8 hours on low, or until the beef is fully cooked and tender.

4. Final Touches:
Stir the mixture well to ensure even distribution of ingredients.
Allow to cool before serving.

PORTION CONTROL AND SIZE RECOMMENDATIONS:

Small Dogs: 1/2 cup per meal
Medium Dogs: 1 cup per meal
Large Dogs: 2 cups per meal

NUTRITIONAL INFORMATION AND CALORIE REQUIREMENTS:

Small Portion (1/2 cup):
Calories: 155 kcal
Protein: 21g
Fat: 6g
Carbohydrates: 9g
Medium Portion (1 cup):
Calories: 310 kcal
Protein: 42g
Fat: 12g
Carbohydrates: 18g
Large Portion (2 cups):
Calories: 620 kcal
Protein: 84g
Fat: 24g
Carbohydrates: 36g

ADAPTATIONS FOR DIFFERENT LIFE STAGES, BREEDS, AND ACTIVITY LEVELS:

Puppies:
Increase protein by adding an extra 1/2 cup of diced beef.
Ensure the mixture is finely chopped for easier digestion.
Adults:
Follow the standard recipe.
Seniors:
Reduce protein slightly by removing 1/2 cup of beef.
Add an extra 1/4 cup of butternut squash for additional fiber.
High-Activity Dogs:
Increase portion size by 25% to meet higher energy needs.
Low-Activity Dogs:
Ensure portion control to prevent weight gain.
Monitor and adjust based on the dog's activity and weight management needs.

HEARTY BEEF AND CARROT SOUP

INGREDIENTS 1 POUND OF BEEF (GROUND OR DICED)

1/2 cup of barley (cooked)

1 cup of celery (chopped)

2 cups of carrots (chopped)

1 teaspoon of thyme

INSTRUCTIONS

1. Preparation:
Wash and chop the celery and carrots.
If using diced beef, cut it into bite-sized pieces.

2. Layering Ingredients:
Add the beef, cooked barley, chopped celery, carrots, and thyme to the slow cooker, layering them evenly.
Add enough water to cover the ingredients.

3. Cooking:
Set the slow cooker to low and cook for 6-8 hours, until the beef is tender and the vegetables are soft.

4. Final Touches:
Allow the soup to cool completely before serving. Store in an airtight container in the refrigerator.

PORTION CONTROL AND SIZE RECOMMENDATIONS: SMALL DOGS (10-20 LBS): 1/2 CUP PER MEAL

Medium Dogs (20-50 lbs): 1 cup per meal
Large Dogs (50+ lbs): 1 1/2 - 2 cups per meal

NUTRITIONAL INFORMATION AND CALORIE REQUIREMENTS:

Small Portion (1/2 cup):
Calories: 80 kcal
Protein: 10g
Fat: 4g
Carbohydrates: 6g

Medium Portion (1 cup):
Calories: 160 kcal
Protein: 20g
Fat: 8g
Carbohydrates: 12g

Large Portion (1 1/2 - 2 cups):
Calories: 240-320 kcal
Protein: 30-40g
Fat: 12-16g
Carbohydrates: 18-24g

ADAPTATIONS FOR DIFFERENT LIFE STAGES, BREEDS, AND ACTIVITY LEVELS:

Puppies:
Increase protein by adding an extra 1/4 cup of beef. Ensure the ingredients are finely chopped or mashed for easier digestion.

Adults:
Follow the standard portion recommendations.

Seniors:
Reduce protein slightly by removing 1/4 cup of beef.
Make sure the soup is soft and easy to chew by cooking the vegetables until very tender.

High-Activity Dogs:
Increase portion size by 25% to meet higher energy needs.

Low-Activity Dogs:
Reduce portion size by 25% to prevent overfeeding.

BEEF AND VEGGIE CASSEROLE

INGREDIENTS

- 2 pounds of beef (ground or diced)
- 1 cup of reduced quinoa (cooked)
- 1 cup of peas
- 1 cup of carrots (chopped)
- 1/2 teaspoon of oregano
- 2 cups of water

INSTRUCTIONS

1. Preparation:
Dice or ground the beef.
Measure out the cooked quinoa.
Chop the carrots.

2. Layering Ingredients:
Place the beef at the bottom of the slow cooker.
Add the quinoa, peas, and carrots on top of the beef.
Sprinkle the oregano over the top.
Pour in the water to ensure the ingredients are well-moistened.

3. Cooking:
Cover the slow cooker with the lid and set it to low heat.
Cook for 6-8 hours on low, or until the beef is fully cooked and tender.

4. Final Touches:
Stir the mixture well to ensure even distribution of ingredients.
Allow to cool before serving.

PORTION CONTROL AND SIZE RECOMMENDATIONS:

Small Dogs: 1/2 cup per meal
Medium Dogs: 1 cup per meal
Large Dogs: 2 cups per meal

NUTRITIONAL INFORMATION AND CALORIE REQUIREMENTS:

Small Portion (1/2 cup):
Calories: 140 kcal
Protein: 19g
Fat: 6g
Carbohydrates: 8g

Medium Portion (1 cup):
Calories: 280 kcal
Protein: 38g
Fat: 12g
Carbohydrates: 16g

Large Portion (2 cups):
Calories: 560 kcal
Protein: 76g
Fat: 24g
Carbohydrates: 32g

ADAPTATIONS FOR DIFFERENT LIFE STAGES, BREEDS, AND ACTIVITY LEVELS:

Puppies:
Increase protein by adding an extra 1/2 cup of diced beef.
Ensure the mixture is finely chopped for easier digestion.

Adults:
Follow the standard recipe.

Seniors:
Reduce protein slightly by removing 1/2 cup of beef.
Add an extra 1/4 cup of quinoa for additional fiber.

High-Activity Dogs:
Increase portion size by 25% to meet higher energy needs.

Low-Activity Dogs:
Ensure portion control to prevent weight gain.
Monitor and adjust based on the dog's activity and weight management needs

BEEF AND APPLE DELIGHT

INGREDIENTS

- 2 pounds of beef (ground or diced)
- 1 cup of apples (diced)
- 1 cup of carrots (chopped)
- 1 cup of spinach (chopped)
- 1/2 teaspoon of ginger
- 2 cups of water

INSTRUCTIONS

1. Preparation:
Dice or ground the beef.
Dice the apples and chop the carrots.
Chop the spinach.

2. Layering Ingredients:
Place the beef at the bottom of the slow cooker.
Add the apples, carrots, and spinach on top of the beef.
Sprinkle the ginger over the top.
Pour in the water to ensure the ingredients are well-moistened.

3. Cooking:
Cover the slow cooker with the lid and set it to low heat.
Cook for 6-8 hours on low, or until the beef is fully cooked and tender.

4. Final Touches:
Stir the mixture well to ensure even distribution of ingredients.
Allow to cool before serving.

PORTION CONTROL AND SIZE RECOMMENDATIONS:

Small Dogs: 1/2 cup per meal
Medium Dogs: 1 cup per meal
Large Dogs: 2 cups per meal

NUTRITIONAL INFORMATION AND CALORIE REQUIREMENTS:

Small Portion (1/2 cup):
Calories: 130 kcal
Protein: 19g
Fat: 5g
Carbohydrates: 7g
Medium Portion (1 cup):
Calories: 260 kcal
Protein: 38g
Fat: 10g
Carbohydrates: 14g
Large Portion (2 cups):
Calories: 520 kcal
Protein: 76g
Fat: 20g
Carbohydrates: 28g

ADAPTATIONS FOR DIFFERENT LIFE STAGES, BREEDS, AND ACTIVITY LEVELS:

Puppies:
Increase protein by adding an extra 1/2 cup of diced beef.
Ensure the mixture is finely chopped for easier digestion.
Adults:
Follow the standard recipe.
Seniors:
Reduce protein slightly by removing 1/2 cup of beef.
Add an extra 1/4 cup of carrots for additional fiber.
High-Activity Dogs:
Increase portion size by 25% to meet higher energy needs.
Low-Activity Dogs:
Ensure portion control to prevent weight gain.
Monitor and adjust based on the dog's activity and weight management needs.

COCONUT BEEF AND VEGGIES

INGREDIENTS

- 2 pounds of beef (ground or diced)
- 1 cup of coconut milk
- 1 cup of green beans (chopped)
- 1 cup of reduced sweet potatoes (cubed)
- 1/2 teaspoon of turmeric
- 2 cups of water

INSTRUCTIONS

1. Preparation:
Dice or ground the beef.
Chop the green beans and cube the sweet potatoes.
Measure out the coconut milk.

2. Layering Ingredients:
Place the beef at the bottom of the slow cooker.
Add the green beans and sweet potatoes on top of the beef.
Sprinkle the turmeric over the top.
Pour in the coconut milk and water to ensure the ingredients are well-moistened.

3. Cooking:
Cover the slow cooker with the lid and set it to low heat.
Cook for 6-8 hours on low, or until the beef is fully cooked and tender.

4. Final Touches:
Stir the mixture well to ensure even distribution of ingredients.
Allow to cool before serving.

PORTION CONTROL AND SIZE RECOMMENDATIONS:

Small Dogs: 1/2 cup per meal
Medium Dogs: 1 cup per meal
Large Dogs: 2 cups per meal

NUTRITIONAL INFORMATION AND CALORIE REQUIREMENTS:

Small Portion (1/2 cup):
Calories: 140 kcal
Protein: 19g
Fat: 6g
Carbohydrates: 7g

Medium Portion (1 cup):
Calories: 280 kcal
Protein: 38g
Fat: 12g
Carbohydrates: 14g

Large Portion (2 cups):
Calories: 560 kcal
Protein: 76g
Fat: 24g
Carbohydrates: 28g

ADAPTATIONS FOR DIFFERENT LIFE STAGES, BREEDS, AND ACTIVITY LEVELS:

Puppies:
Increase protein by adding an extra 1/2 cup of diced beef.
Ensure the mixture is finely chopped for easier digestion.

Adults:
Follow the standard recipe.

Seniors:
Reduce protein slightly by removing 1/2 cup of beef.
Add an extra 1/4 cup of green beans for additional fiber.

High-Activity Dogs:
Increase portion size by 25% to meet higher energy needs.

Low-Activity Dogs:
Ensure portion control to prevent weight gain.
Monitor and adjust based on the dog's activity and weight management needs.

BEEF AND PEAR COMBO

INGREDIENTS

- 2 pounds of beef (ground or diced)
- 1 cup of pears (diced)
- 1 cup of spinach (chopped)
- 1 cup of cauliflower rice
- 1/2 teaspoon of dill
- 2 cups of water

INSTRUCTIONS

1. Preparation:
Dice or ground the beef.
Dice the pears and chop the spinach.

2. Layering Ingredients:
Place the beef at the bottom of the slow cooker.
Add the pears, spinach, and cauliflower rice on top of the beef.
Sprinkle the dill over the top.
Pour in the water to ensure the ingredients are well-moistened.

3. Cooking:
Cover the slow cooker with the lid and set it to low heat.
Cook for 6-8 hours on low, or until the beef is fully cooked and tender.

4. Final Touches:
Stir the mixture well to ensure even distribution of ingredients.
Allow to cool before serving.

PORTION CONTROL AND SIZE RECOMMENDATIONS:

Small Dogs: 1/2 cup per meal
Medium Dogs: 1 cup per meal
Large Dogs: 2 cups per meal

NUTRITIONAL INFORMATION AND CALORIE REQUIREMENTS:

Small Portion (1/2 cup):
Calories: 120 kcal
Protein: 18g
Fat: 5g
Carbohydrates: 6g

Medium Portion (1 cup):
Calories: 240 kcal
Protein: 36g
Fat: 10g
Carbohydrates: 12g

Large Portion (2 cups):
Calories: 480 kcal
Protein: 72g
Fat: 20g
Carbohydrates: 24g

ADAPTATIONS FOR DIFFERENT LIFE STAGES, BREEDS, AND ACTIVITY LEVELS:

Puppies:
Increase protein by adding an extra 1/2 cup of diced beef.
Ensure the mixture is finely chopped for easier digestion.

Adults:
Follow the standard recipe.

Seniors:
Reduce protein slightly by removing 1/2 cup of beef.
Add an extra 1/4 cup of spinach for additional fiber.

High-Activity Dogs:
Increase portion size by 25% to meet higher energy needs.

Low-Activity Dogs:
Ensure portion control to prevent weight gain.
Monitor and adjust based on the dog's activity and weight management needs.

BEEF AND SPINACH DELIGHT

INGREDIENTS

- 2 pounds of beef (ground or diced)
- 1 cup of cauliflower rice
- 1 cup of carrots (chopped)
- 1 cup of spinach (chopped)
- 1/2 teaspoon of basil
- 2 cups of water

INSTRUCTIONS

1. Preparation:
Dice or ground the beef.
Chop the carrots and spinach.
Measure out the cauliflower rice.

2. Layering Ingredients:
Place the beef at the bottom of the slow cooker.
Add the cauliflower rice, carrots, and spinach on top of the beef.
Sprinkle the basil over the top.
Pour in the water to ensure the ingredients are well-moistened.

3. Cooking:
Cover the slow cooker with the lid and set it to low heat.
Cook for 6-8 hours on low, or until the beef is fully cooked and tender.

4. Final Touches:
Stir the mixture well to ensure even distribution of ingredients.
Allow to cool before serving.

PORTION CONTROL AND SIZE RECOMMENDATIONS:

Small Dogs: 1/2 cup per meal
Medium Dogs: 1 cup per meal
Large Dogs: 2 cups per meal

NUTRITIONAL INFORMATION AND CALORIE REQUIREMENTS:

Small Portion (1/2 cup):
Calories: 130 kcal
Protein: 19g
Fat: 6g
Carbohydrates: 5g
Medium Portion (1 cup):
Calories: 260 kcal
Protein: 38g
Fat: 12g
Carbohydrates: 10g
Large Portion (2 cups):
Calories: 520 kcal
Protein: 76g
Fat: 24g
Carbohydrates: 20g

ADAPTATIONS FOR DIFFERENT LIFE STAGES, BREEDS, AND ACTIVITY LEVELS:

Puppies:
Increase protein by adding an extra 1/2 cup of diced beef.
Ensure the mixture is finely chopped for easier digestion.
Adults:
Follow the standard recipe.
Seniors:
Reduce protein slightly by removing 1/2 cup of beef.
Add an extra 1/4 cup of carrots for additional fiber.
High-Activity Dogs:
Increase portion size by 25% to meet higher energy needs.
Low-Activity Dogs:
Ensure portion control to prevent weight gain.
Monitor and adjust based on the dog's activity and weight management needs.

BEEF AND TURNIP STEW

INGREDIENTS

- 2 pounds of beef (ground or diced)
- 1 cup of turnips (chopped)
- 1 cup of green beans (chopped)
- 1 cup of reduced quinoa
- 1/2 teaspoon of rosemary
- 2 cups of water

INSTRUCTIONS

1. Preparation:
Dice or ground the beef.
Chop the turnips and green beans.
Measure out the reduced quinoa.

2. Layering Ingredients:
Place the beef at the bottom of the slow cooker.
Add the turnips, green beans, and quinoa on top of the beef.
Sprinkle the rosemary over the top.
Pour in the water to ensure the ingredients are well-moistened.

3. Cooking:
Cover the slow cooker with the lid and set it to low heat.
Cook for 6-8 hours on low, or until the beef is fully cooked and tender.

4. Final Touches:
Stir the mixture well to ensure even distribution of ingredients.
Allow to cool before serving.

PORTION CONTROL AND SIZE RECOMMENDATIONS:

Small Dogs: 1/2 cup per meal
Medium Dogs: 1 cup per meal
Large Dogs: 2 cups per meal

NUTRITIONAL INFORMATION AND CALORIE REQUIREMENTS:

Small Portion (1/2 cup):
Calories: 150 kcal
Protein: 20g
Fat: 7g
Carbohydrates: 8g
Medium Portion (1 cup):
Calories: 300 kcal
Protein: 40g
Fat: 14g
Carbohydrates: 16g
Large Portion (2 cups):
Calories: 600 kcal
Protein: 80g
Fat: 28g
Carbohydrates: 32g

ADAPTATIONS FOR DIFFERENT LIFE STAGES, BREEDS, AND ACTIVITY LEVELS:

Puppies:
Increase protein by adding an extra 1/2 cup of diced beef.
Ensure the mixture is finely chopped for easier digestion.
Adults:
Follow the standard recipe.
Seniors:
Reduce protein slightly by removing 1/2 cup of beef.
Add an extra 1/4 cup of turnips for additional fiber.
High-Activity Dogs:
Increase portion size by 25% to meet higher energy needs.
Low-Activity Dogs:
Ensure portion control to prevent weight gain.
Monitor and adjust based on the dog's activity and weight management needs.

LAMB AND PUMPKIN BLEND

INGREDIENTS

- 2 pounds of lean lamb (boneless)
- 1 cup of pumpkin (chopped)
- 1 cup of kale (chopped)
- 1 cup of apples (cored and chopped)
- 1/2 teaspoon of ginger (ground)

INSTRUCTIONS

1. Preparation:
Wash and chop all vegetables and fruits.
Chop the lamb into bite-sized pieces.

2. Layering Ingredients:
Place the lamb pieces at the bottom of the slow cooker.
Add the chopped pumpkin, kale, and apples.
Sprinkle the ginger on top.

3. Cooking:
Cover the slow cooker with the lid.
Set the slow cooker to low heat and cook for 6-8 hours, or until the lamb is fully cooked and tender.

4. Final Touches:
Stir the mixture well to ensure even distribution of ingredients.
Allow to cool before serving.

PORTION CONTROL AND SIZE RECOMMENDATIONS:

Small Dogs (10-20 lbs): 1/2 cup per meal
Medium Dogs (20-50 lbs): 1 cup per meal
Large Dogs (50+ lbs): 1 1/2 - 2 cups per meal

NUTRITIONAL INFORMATION AND CALORIE REQUIREMENTS:

Small Portion (1/2 cup):
Calories: 180 kcal
Protein: 15g
Fat: 8g
Carbohydrates: 10g

Medium Portion (1 cup):
Calories: 360 kcal
Protein: 30g
Fat: 16g
Carbohydrates: 20g

Large Portion (2 cups):
Calories: 720 kcal
Protein: 60g
Fat: 32g
Carbohydrates: 40g

ADAPTATIONS FOR DIFFERENT LIFE STAGES, BREEDS, AND ACTIVITY LEVELS:

Puppies:
Increase protein by adding an extra 1/4 cup of chopped lamb.
Ensure the mixture is finely chopped for easier digestion.

Adults:
Follow the standard recipe.

Seniors:
Reduce protein slightly by removing 1/4 cup of lamb.
Add an extra 1/4 cup of chopped kale for additional fiber.

High-Activity Dogs:
Increase portion size by 25% to meet higher energy needs.

Low-Activity Dogs:
Reduce portion size by 25% to prevent overfeeding.

HERBED LAMB AND VEGGIES

INGREDIENTS

- 2 pounds of lean lamb (boneless)
- 1 teaspoon of rosemary
- 1 cup of peas
- 1 cup of zucchini (chopped)
- 1 tablespoon of parsley (chopped)

INSTRUCTIONS

1. Preparation:
Wash and chop all vegetables.
Chop the lamb into bite-sized pieces.

2. Layering Ingredients:
Place the lamb pieces at the bottom of the slow cooker.
Add the peas and chopped zucchini.
Sprinkle the rosemary and chopped parsley on top.

3. Cooking:
Cover the slow cooker with the lid.
Set the slow cooker to low heat and cook for 6-8 hours, or until the lamb is fully cooked and tender.

4. Final Touches:
Stir the mixture well to ensure even distribution of ingredients.
Allow to cool before serving.

PORTION CONTROL AND SIZE RECOMMENDATIONS:

Small Dogs (10-20 lbs): 1/2 cup per meal
Medium Dogs (20-50 lbs): 1 cup per meal
Large Dogs (50+ lbs): 1 1/2 - 2 cups per meal

NUTRITIONAL INFORMATION AND CALORIE REQUIREMENTS:

Small Portion (1/2 cup):
Calories: 175 kcal
Protein: 14g
Fat: 8g
Carbohydrates: 9g

Medium Portion (1 cup):
Calories: 350 kcal
Protein: 28g
Fat: 16g
Carbohydrates: 18g

Large Portion (2 cups):
Calories: 700 kcal
Protein: 56g
Fat: 32g
Carbohydrates: 36g

ADAPTATIONS FOR DIFFERENT LIFE STAGES, BREEDS, AND ACTIVITY LEVELS:

Puppies:
Increase protein by adding an extra 1/4 cup of chopped lamb.
Ensure the mixture is finely chopped for easier digestion.

Adults:
Follow the standard recipe.

Seniors:
Reduce protein slightly by removing 1/4 cup of lamb.
Add an extra 1/4 cup of chopped peas for additional fiber.

High-Activity Dogs:
Increase portion size by 25% to meet higher energy needs.

Low-Activity Dogs:
Reduce portion size by 25% to prevent overfeeding.

LAMB AND SPINACH DELIGHT

INGREDIENTS

- 2 pounds of lean lamb (boneless)
- 1 cup of cauliflower rice
- 1 cup of carrots (chopped)
- 1 cup of spinach (chopped)
- 1/2 teaspoon of basil

INSTRUCTIONS

1. Preparation:
Wash and chop all vegetables.
Chop the lamb into bite-sized pieces.

2. Layering Ingredients:
Place the lamb pieces at the bottom of the slow cooker.
Add the cauliflower rice, chopped carrots, and spinach.
Sprinkle the basil on top.

3. Cooking:
Cover the slow cooker with the lid.
Set the slow cooker to low heat and cook for 6-8 hours, or until the lamb is fully cooked and tender.

4. Final Touches:
Stir the mixture well to ensure even distribution of ingredients.
Allow to cool before serving.

PORTION CONTROL AND SIZE RECOMMENDATIONS:

Small Dogs (10-20 lbs): 1/2 cup per meal
Medium Dogs (20-50 lbs): 1 cup per meal
Large Dogs (50+ lbs): 1 1/2 - 2 cups per meal

NUTRITIONAL INFORMATION AND CALORIE REQUIREMENTS:

Small Portion (1/2 cup):
Calories: 170 kcal
Protein: 14g
Fat: 7g
Carbohydrates: 10g

Medium Portion (1 cup):
Calories: 340 kcal
Protein: 28g
Fat: 14g
Carbohydrates: 20g

Large Portion (2 cups):
Calories: 680 kcal
Protein: 56g
Fat: 28g
Carbohydrates: 40g

ADAPTATIONS FOR DIFFERENT LIFE STAGES, BREEDS, AND ACTIVITY LEVELS:

Puppies:
Increase protein by adding an extra 1/4 cup of chopped lamb.
Ensure the mixture is finely chopped for easier digestion.

Adults:
Follow the standard recipe.

Seniors:
Reduce protein slightly by removing 1/4 cup of lamb.
Add an extra 1/4 cup of chopped spinach for additional fiber.

High-Activity Dogs:
Increase portion size by 25% to meet higher energy needs.

Low-Activity Dogs:
Reduce portion size by 25% to prevent overfeeding.

LAMB AND LENTIL SOUP

INGREDIENTS

- 2 pounds of lean lamb (boneless)
- 1 cup of reduced lentils
- 1 cup of carrots (chopped)
- 1 cup of green beans (chopped)
- 1/2 teaspoon of turmeric

INSTRUCTIONS

1. Preparation:
Wash and chop all vegetables.
Rinse and reduce the lentils as per package instructions.
Chop the lamb into bite-sized pieces.

2. Layering Ingredients:
Place the lamb pieces at the bottom of the slow cooker.
Add the reduced lentils, chopped carrots, and green beans.
Sprinkle the turmeric on top.

3. Cooking:
Cover the slow cooker with the lid.
Set the slow cooker to low heat and cook for 6-8 hours, or until the lamb is fully cooked and the lentils are tender.

4. Final Touches:
Stir the mixture well to ensure even distribution of ingredients.
Allow to cool before serving.

PORTION CONTROL AND SIZE RECOMMENDATIONS:

Small Dogs (10-20 lbs): 1/2 cup per meal
Medium Dogs (20-50 lbs): 1 cup per meal
Large Dogs (50+ lbs): 1 1/2 - 2 cups per meal

NUTRITIONAL INFORMATION AND CALORIE REQUIREMENTS:

Small Portion (1/2 cup):
Calories: 180 kcal
Protein: 15g
Fat: 8g
Carbohydrates: 10g
Medium Portion (1 cup):
Calories: 360 kcal
Protein: 30g
Fat: 16g
Carbohydrates: 20g
Large Portion (2 cups):
Calories: 720 kcal
Protein: 60g
Fat: 32g
Carbohydrates: 40g

ADAPTATIONS FOR DIFFERENT LIFE STAGES, BREEDS, AND ACTIVITY LEVELS:

Puppies:
Increase protein by adding an extra 1/4 cup of chopped lamb.
Ensure the mixture is finely chopped for easier digestion.
Adults:
Follow the standard recipe.
Seniors:
Reduce protein slightly by removing 1/4 cup of lamb.
Add an extra 1/4 cup of chopped green beans for additional fiber.
High-Activity Dogs:
Increase portion size by 25% to meet higher energy needs.
Low-Activity Dogs:
Reduce portion size by 25% to prevent overfeeding.

LAMB AND SWEET POTATO DELIGHT

INGREDIENTS

- 2 pounds of lean lamb (boneless)
- 1 cup of reduced sweet potatoes (chopped)
- 1 cup of broccoli (chopped)
- 1 teaspoon of rosemary
- 1/2 teaspoon of turmeric

INSTRUCTIONS

1. Preparation:
Wash and chop all vegetables.
Rinse and reduce the sweet potatoes as per package instructions.
Chop the lamb into bite-sized pieces.

2. Layering Ingredients:
Place the lamb pieces at the bottom of the slow cooker.
Add the reduced sweet potatoes and chopped broccoli.
Sprinkle the rosemary and turmeric on top.

3. Cooking:
Cover the slow cooker with the lid.
Set the slow cooker to low heat and cook for 6-8 hours, or until the lamb is fully cooked and the vegetables are tender.

4. Final Touches:
Stir the mixture well to ensure even distribution of ingredients.
Allow to cool before serving.

PORTION CONTROL AND SIZE RECOMMENDATIONS:

Small Dogs (10-20 lbs): 1/2 cup per meal
Medium Dogs (20-50 lbs): 1 cup per meal
Large Dogs (50+ lbs): 1 1/2 - 2 cups per meal

NUTRITIONAL INFORMATION AND CALORIE REQUIREMENTS:

Small Portion (1/2 cup):
Calories: 185 kcal
Protein: 16g
Fat: 7g
Carbohydrates: 12g
Medium Portion (1 cup):
Calories: 370 kcal
Protein: 32g
Fat: 14g
Carbohydrates: 24g
Large Portion (2 cups):
Calories: 740 kcal
Protein: 64g
Fat: 28g
Carbohydrates: 48g

ADAPTATIONS FOR DIFFERENT LIFE STAGES, BREEDS, AND ACTIVITY LEVELS:

Puppies:
Increase protein by adding an extra 1/4 cup of chopped lamb.
Ensure the mixture is finely chopped for easier digestion.
Adults:
Follow the standard recipe.
Seniors:
Reduce protein slightly by removing 1/4 cup of lamb.
Add an extra 1/4 cup of chopped broccoli for additional fiber.
High-Activity Dogs:
Increase portion size by 25% to meet higher energy needs.
Low-Activity Dogs:
Reduce portion size by 25% to prevent overfeeding.

LAMB AND APPLE DELIGHT

INGREDIENTS

- 2 pounds of lean lamb (boneless)
- 1 cup of apples (cored and chopped)
- 1 cup of carrots (chopped)
- 1 cup of cauliflower rice
- 1/2 teaspoon of ginger

INSTRUCTIONS

1. Preparation:

Wash and chop all vegetables and fruits.
Chop the lamb into bite-sized pieces.

2. Layering Ingredients:

Place the lamb pieces at the bottom of the slow cooker.
Add the chopped apples, carrots, and cauliflower rice.
Sprinkle the ginger on top.

3. Cooking:

Cover the slow cooker with the lid.
Set the slow cooker to low heat and cook for 6-8 hours, or until the lamb is fully cooked and the vegetables are tender.

4. Final Touches:

Stir the mixture well to ensure even distribution of ingredients.
Allow to cool before serving.

PORTION CONTROL AND SIZE RECOMMENDATIONS:

Small Dogs (10-20 lbs): 1/2 cup per meal
Medium Dogs (20-50 lbs): 1 cup per meal
Large Dogs (50+ lbs): 1 1/2 - 2 cups per meal

NUTRITIONAL INFORMATION AND CALORIE REQUIREMENTS:

Small Portion (1/2 cup):
Calories: 170 kcal
Protein: 14g
Fat: 8g
Carbohydrates: 9g

Medium Portion (1 cup):
Calories: 340 kcal
Protein: 28g
Fat: 16g
Carbohydrates: 18g

Large Portion (2 cups):
Calories: 680 kcal
Protein: 56g
Fat: 32g
Carbohydrates: 36g

ADAPTATIONS FOR DIFFERENT LIFE STAGES, BREEDS, AND ACTIVITY LEVELS:

Puppies:
Increase protein by adding an extra 1/4 cup of chopped lamb.
Ensure the mixture is finely chopped for easier digestion.

Adults:
Follow the standard recipe.

Seniors:
Reduce protein slightly by removing 1/4 cup of lamb.
Add an extra 1/4 cup of chopped cauliflower rice for additional fiber.

High-Activity Dogs:
Increase portion size by 25% to meet higher energy needs.

Low-Activity Dogs:
Reduce portion size by 25% to prevent overfeeding.

LAMB AND VEGGIE CASSEROLE

INGREDIENTS

- 2 pounds of lean lamb (boneless)
- 1 cup of reduced barley
- 1 cup of carrots (chopped)
- 1 cup of green beans (chopped)
- 1/2 teaspoon of thyme

INSTRUCTIONS

1. Preparation:

Wash and chop all vegetables.

Rinse and reduce the barley as per package instructions.

Chop the lamb into bite-sized pieces.

2. Layering Ingredients:

Place the lamb pieces at the bottom of the slow cooker.

Add the reduced barley, chopped carrots, and green beans.

Sprinkle the thyme on top.

3. Cooking:

Cover the slow cooker with the lid.

Set the slow cooker to low heat and cook for 6-8 hours, or until the lamb is fully cooked and the barley is tender.

4. Final Touches:

Stir the mixture well to ensure even distribution of ingredients.

Allow to cool before serving.

PORTION CONTROL AND SIZE RECOMMENDATIONS:

Small Dogs (10-20 lbs): 1/2 cup per meal
Medium Dogs (20-50 lbs): 1 cup per meal
Large Dogs (50+ lbs): 1 1/2 - 2 cups per meal

NUTRITIONAL INFORMATION AND CALORIE REQUIREMENTS:

Small Portion (1/2 cup):
Calories: 175 kcal
Protein: 14g
Fat: 7g
Carbohydrates: 9g
Medium Portion (1 cup):
Calories: 350 kcal
Protein: 28g
Fat: 14g
Carbohydrates: 18g
Large Portion (2 cups):
Calories: 700 kcal
Protein: 56g
Fat: 28g
Carbohydrates: 36g

ADAPTATIONS FOR DIFFERENT LIFE STAGES, BREEDS, AND ACTIVITY LEVELS:

Puppies:
Increase protein by adding an extra 1/4 cup of chopped lamb.
Ensure the mixture is finely chopped for easier digestion.
Adults:
Follow the standard recipe.
Seniors:
Reduce protein slightly by removing 1/4 cup of lamb.
Add an extra 1/4 cup of chopped carrots for additional fiber.
High-Activity Dogs:
Increase portion size by 25% to meet higher energy needs.
Low-Activity Dogs:
Reduce portion size by 25% to prevent overfeeding.

LAMB AND MINT STEW

INGREDIENTS

- 2 pounds of lean lamb (boneless)
- 1 tablespoon of fresh mint (chopped)
- 1 cup of peas
- 1 cup of reduced sweet potatoes (chopped)
- 1/2 teaspoon of dill

INSTRUCTIONS

1. Preparation:
Wash and chop all vegetables.
Rinse and reduce the sweet potatoes as per package instructions.
Chop the lamb into bite-sized pieces.

2. Layering Ingredients:
Place the lamb pieces at the bottom of the slow cooker.
Add the peas and reduced sweet potatoes.
Sprinkle the chopped mint and dill on top.

3. Cooking:
Cover the slow cooker with the lid.
Set the slow cooker to low heat and cook for 6-8 hours, or until the lamb is fully cooked and the vegetables are tender.

4. Final Touches:
Stir the mixture well to ensure even distribution of ingredients.
Allow to cool before serving.

PORTION CONTROL AND SIZE RECOMMENDATIONS:

Small Dogs (10-20 lbs): 1/2 cup per meal
Medium Dogs (20-50 lbs): 1 cup per meal
Large Dogs (50+ lbs): 1 1/2 - 2 cups per meal

NUTRITIONAL INFORMATION AND CALORIE REQUIREMENTS:

Small Portion (1/2 cup):
Calories: 180 kcal
Protein: 15g
Fat: 8g
Carbohydrates: 10g

Medium Portion (1 cup):
Calories: 360 kcal
Protein: 30g
Fat: 16g
Carbohydrates: 20g

Large Portion (2 cups):
Calories: 720 kcal
Protein: 60g
Fat: 32g
Carbohydrates: 40g

ADAPTATIONS FOR DIFFERENT LIFE STAGES, BREEDS, AND ACTIVITY LEVELS:

Puppies:
Increase protein by adding an extra 1/4 cup of chopped lamb.
Ensure the mixture is finely chopped for easier digestion.

Adults:
Follow the standard recipe.

Seniors:
Reduce protein slightly by removing 1/4 cup of lamb.
Add an extra 1/4 cup of peas for additional fiber.

High-Activity Dogs:
Increase portion size by 25% to meet higher energy needs.

Low-Activity Dogs:
Reduce portion size by 25% to prevent overfeeding.

LAMB AND CHICKPEA STEW

INGREDIENTS

- 2 pounds of lean lamb (boneless)
- 1 cup of reduced chickpeas
- 1 cup of spinach (chopped)
- 1 tablespoon of parsley (chopped)
- 1/2 teaspoon of cumin

INSTRUCTIONS

1. Preparation:
Wash and chop all vegetables.
Rinse and reduce the chickpeas as per package instructions.
Chop the lamb into bite-sized pieces.

2. Layering Ingredients:
Place the lamb pieces at the bottom of the slow cooker.
Add the reduced chickpeas and chopped spinach.
Sprinkle the chopped parsley and cumin on top.

3. Cooking:
Cover the slow cooker with the lid.
Set the slow cooker to low heat and cook for 6-8 hours, or until the lamb is fully cooked and the chickpeas are tender.

4. Final Touches:
Stir the mixture well to ensure even distribution of ingredients.
Allow to cool before serving.

PORTION CONTROL AND SIZE RECOMMENDATIONS:

Small Dogs (10-20 lbs): 1/2 cup per meal
Medium Dogs (20-50 lbs): 1 cup per meal
Large Dogs (50+ lbs): 1 1/2 - 2 cups per meal

NUTRITIONAL INFORMATION AND CALORIE REQUIREMENTS:

Small Portion (1/2 cup):
Calories: 185 kcal
Protein: 15g
Fat: 9g
Carbohydrates: 10g
Medium Portion (1 cup):
Calories: 370 kcal
Protein: 30g
Fat: 18g
Carbohydrates: 20g
Large Portion (2 cups):
Calories: 740 kcal
Protein: 60g
Fat: 36g
Carbohydrates: 40g

ADAPTATIONS FOR DIFFERENT LIFE STAGES, BREEDS, AND ACTIVITY LEVELS:

Puppies:
Increase protein by adding an extra 1/4 cup of chopped lamb.
Ensure the mixture is finely chopped for easier digestion.
Adults:
Follow the standard recipe.
Seniors:
Reduce protein slightly by removing 1/4 cup of lamb.
Add an extra 1/4 cup of chopped spinach for additional fiber.
High-Activity Dogs:
Increase portion size by 25% to meet higher energy needs.
Low-Activity Dogs:
Reduce portion size by 25% to prevent overfeeding.

LAMB AND VEGGIE MIX

INGREDIENTS

- 2 pounds of lean lamb (boneless)
- 1 cup of reduced quinoa
- 1 cup of spinach (chopped)
- 1 cup of sweet corn
- 1/2 teaspoon of oregano

INSTRUCTIONS

1. Preparation:
Wash and chop all vegetables.
Rinse and reduce the quinoa as per package instructions.
Chop the lamb into bite-sized pieces.

2. Layering Ingredients:
Place the lamb pieces at the bottom of the slow cooker.
Add the reduced quinoa, chopped spinach, and sweet corn.
Sprinkle the oregano on top.

3. Cooking:
Cover the slow cooker with the lid.
Set the slow cooker to low heat and cook for 6-8 hours, or until the lamb is fully cooked and the quinoa is tender.

4. Final Touches:
Stir the mixture well to ensure even distribution of ingredients.
Allow to cool before serving.

PORTION CONTROL AND SIZE RECOMMENDATIONS:

Small Dogs (10-20 lbs): 1/2 cup per meal
Medium Dogs (20-50 lbs): 1 cup per meal
Large Dogs (50+ lbs): 1 1/2 - 2 cups per meal

NUTRITIONAL INFORMATION AND CALORIE REQUIREMENTS:

Small Portion (1/2 cup):
Calories: 175 kcal
Protein: 14g
Fat: 7g
Carbohydrates: 10g

Medium Portion (1 cup):
Calories: 350 kcal
Protein: 28g
Fat: 14g
Carbohydrates: 20g

Large Portion (2 cups):
Calories: 700 kcal
Protein: 56g
Fat: 28g
Carbohydrates: 40g

ADAPTATIONS FOR DIFFERENT LIFE STAGES, BREEDS, AND ACTIVITY LEVELS:

Puppies:
Increase protein by adding an extra 1/4 cup of chopped lamb.
Ensure the mixture is finely chopped for easier digestion.

Adults:
Follow the standard recipe.

Seniors:
Reduce protein slightly by removing 1/4 cup of lamb.
Add an extra 1/4 cup of chopped spinach for additional fiber.

High-Activity Dogs:
Increase portion size by 25% to meet higher energy needs.

Low-Activity Dogs:
Reduce portion size by 25% to prevent overfeeding.

FISH AND BLUEBERRY NUTRIENT BOOST

INGREDIENTS

- 2 pounds of salmon (boneless, skinless)
- 1 cup of blueberries
- 1 cup of spinach (chopped)
- 1 cup of reduced quinoa
- 1/2 teaspoon of basil

INSTRUCTIONS

1. Preparation:
Wash and chop all vegetables.
Rinse and reduce the quinoa as per package instructions.
Chop the salmon into bite-sized pieces.

2. Layering Ingredients:
Place the salmon pieces at the bottom of the slow cooker.
Add the blueberries, chopped spinach, and reduced quinoa.
Sprinkle the basil on top.

3. Cooking:
Cover the slow cooker with the lid.
Set the slow cooker to low heat and cook for 6-8 hours, or until the salmon is fully cooked and the quinoa is tender.

4. Final Touches:
Stir the mixture well to ensure even distribution of ingredients.
Allow to cool before serving.

PORTION CONTROL AND SIZE RECOMMENDATIONS:

Small Dogs (10-20 lbs): 1/2 cup per meal
Medium Dogs (20-50 lbs): 1 cup per meal
Large Dogs (50+ lbs): 1 1/2 - 2 cups per meal

NUTRITIONAL INFORMATION AND CALORIE REQUIREMENTS:

Small Portion (1/2 cup):
Calories: 170 kcal
Protein: 15g
Fat: 8g
Carbohydrates: 8g

Medium Portion (1 cup):
Calories: 340 kcal
Protein: 30g
Fat: 16g
Carbohydrates: 16g

Large Portion (2 cups):
Calories: 680 kcal
Protein: 60g
Fat: 32g
Carbohydrates: 32g

ADAPTATIONS FOR DIFFERENT LIFE STAGES, BREEDS, AND ACTIVITY LEVELS:

Puppies:
Increase protein by adding an extra 1/4 cup of chopped salmon.
Ensure the mixture is finely chopped for easier digestion.

Adults:
Follow the standard recipe.

Seniors:
Reduce protein slightly by removing 1/4 cup of salmon.
Add an extra 1/4 cup of chopped spinach for additional fiber.

High-Activity Dogs:
Increase portion size by 25% to meet higher energy needs.

Low-Activity Dogs:
Reduce portion size by 25% to prevent overfeeding.

SAVORY FISH AND ZUCCHINI MIX

INGREDIENTS

- 2 pounds of cod (boneless, skinless)
- 1 cup of reduced quinoa
- 1 cup of zucchini (chopped)
- 1/2 teaspoon of turmeric
- 1 tablespoon of parsley (chopped)

INSTRUCTIONS

1. Preparation:
Wash and chop all vegetables.
Rinse and reduce the quinoa as per package instructions.
Chop the cod into bite-sized pieces.

2. Layering Ingredients:
Place the cod pieces at the bottom of the slow cooker.
Add the reduced quinoa and chopped zucchini.
Sprinkle the turmeric and chopped parsley on top.

3. Cooking:
Cover the slow cooker with the lid.
Set the slow cooker to low heat and cook for 6-8 hours, or until the cod is fully cooked and the quinoa is tender.

4. Final Touches:
Stir the mixture well to ensure even distribution of ingredients.
Allow to cool before serving.

PORTION CONTROL AND SIZE RECOMMENDATIONS:

Small Dogs (10-20 lbs): 1/2 cup per meal
Medium Dogs (20-50 lbs): 1 cup per meal
Large Dogs (50+ lbs): 1 1/2 - 2 cups per meal

NUTRITIONAL INFORMATION AND CALORIE REQUIREMENTS:

Small Portion (1/2 cup):
Calories: 160 kcal
Protein: 14g
Fat: 6g
Carbohydrates: 9g

Medium Portion (1 cup):
Calories: 320 kcal
Protein: 28g
Fat: 12g
Carbohydrates: 18g

Large Portion (2 cups):
Calories: 640 kcal
Protein: 56g
Fat: 24g
Carbohydrates: 36g

ADAPTATIONS FOR DIFFERENT LIFE STAGES, BREEDS, AND ACTIVITY LEVELS:

Puppies:
Increase protein by adding an extra 1/4 cup of chopped cod.
Ensure the mixture is finely chopped for easier digestion.

Adults:
Follow the standard recipe.

Seniors:
Reduce protein slightly by removing 1/4 cup of cod.
Add an extra 1/4 cup of chopped zucchini for additional fiber.

High-Activity Dogs:
Increase portion size by 25% to meet higher energy needs.

Low-Activity Dogs:
Reduce portion size by 25% to prevent overfeeding.

FISH AND BROCCOLI BLEND

INGREDIENTS

- 2 pounds of salmon (boneless, skinless)
- 1 cup of broccoli (chopped)
- 1 cup of sweet peas
- 1 tablespoon of olive oil
- 1/2 teaspoon of dill

INSTRUCTIONS

1. Preparation:
Wash and chop all vegetables.
Chop the salmon into bite-sized pieces.

2. Layering Ingredients:
Place the salmon pieces at the bottom of the slow cooker.
Add the chopped broccoli and sweet peas.
Drizzle the olive oil and sprinkle the dill on top.

3. Cooking:
Cover the slow cooker with the lid.
Set the slow cooker to low heat and cook for 6-8 hours, or until the salmon is fully cooked and the vegetables are tender.

4. Final Touches:
Stir the mixture well to ensure even distribution of ingredients.
Allow to cool before serving.

PORTION CONTROL AND SIZE RECOMMENDATIONS:

Small Dogs (10-20 lbs): 1/2 cup per meal
Medium Dogs (20-50 lbs): 1 cup per meal
Large Dogs (50+ lbs): 1 1/2 - 2 cups per meal

NUTRITIONAL INFORMATION AND CALORIE REQUIREMENTS:

Small Portion (1/2 cup):
Calories: 170 kcal
Protein: 15g
Fat: 8g
Carbohydrates: 7g

Medium Portion (1 cup):
Calories: 340 kcal
Protein: 30g
Fat: 16g
Carbohydrates: 14g

Large Portion (2 cups):
Calories: 680 kcal
Protein: 60g
Fat: 32g
Carbohydrates: 28g

ADAPTATIONS FOR DIFFERENT LIFE STAGES, BREEDS, AND ACTIVITY LEVELS:

Puppies:
Increase protein by adding an extra 1/4 cup of chopped salmon.
Ensure the mixture is finely chopped for easier digestion.

Adults:
Follow the standard recipe.

Seniors:
Reduce protein slightly by removing 1/4 cup of salmon.
Add an extra 1/4 cup of broccoli for additional fiber.

High-Activity Dogs:
Increase portion size by 25% to meet higher energy needs.

Low-Activity Dogs:
Reduce portion size by 25% to prevent overfeeding.

FISH AND PUMPKIN FEAST

INGREDIENTS

- 2 pounds of salmon (boneless, skinless)
- 1 cup of pumpkin (chopped)
- 1 cup of apples (cored and chopped)
- 1 cup of kale (chopped)
- 1/2 teaspoon of ginger (ground)

INSTRUCTIONS

1. Preparation:
Wash and chop all vegetables and fruits.
Chop the salmon into bite-sized pieces.

2. Layering Ingredients:
Place the salmon pieces at the bottom of the slow cooker.
Add the chopped pumpkin, apples, and kale.
Sprinkle the ginger on top.

3. Cooking:
Cover the slow cooker with the lid.
Set the slow cooker to low heat and cook for 6-8 hours, or until the salmon is fully cooked and the vegetables are tender.

4. Final Touches:
Stir the mixture well to ensure even distribution of ingredients.
Allow to cool before serving.

PORTION CONTROL AND SIZE RECOMMENDATIONS:

Small Dogs (10-20 lbs): 1/2 cup per meal
Medium Dogs (20-50 lbs): 1 cup per meal
Large Dogs (50+ lbs): 1 1/2 - 2 cups per meal

NUTRITIONAL INFORMATION AND CALORIE REQUIREMENTS:

Small Portion (1/2 cup):
Calories: 175 kcal
Protein: 14g
Fat: 7g
Carbohydrates: 10g

Medium Portion (1 cup):
Calories: 350 kcal
Protein: 28g
Fat: 14g
Carbohydrates: 20g

Large Portion (2 cups):
Calories: 700 kcal
Protein: 56g
Fat: 28g
Carbohydrates: 40g

ADAPTATIONS FOR DIFFERENT LIFE STAGES, BREEDS, AND ACTIVITY LEVELS:

Puppies:
Increase protein by adding an extra 1/4 cup of chopped salmon.
Ensure the mixture is finely chopped for easier digestion.

Adults:
Follow the standard recipe.

Seniors:
Reduce protein slightly by removing 1/4 cup of salmon.
Add an extra 1/4 cup of pumpkin for additional fiber.

High-Activity Dogs:
Increase portion size by 25% to meet higher energy needs.

Low-Activity Dogs:
Reduce portion size by 25% to prevent overfeeding.

FISH AND SWEET POTATO DELIGHT

INGREDIENTS

- 2 pounds of cod (boneless, skinless)
- 1 cup of reduced sweet potatoes (chopped)
- 1 cup of spinach (chopped)
- 1/2 teaspoon of dill
- 1 tablespoon of lemon juice

INSTRUCTIONS

1. Preparation:
Wash and chop all vegetables.
Rinse and reduce the sweet potatoes as per package instructions.
Chop the cod into bite-sized pieces.

2. Layering Ingredients:
Place the cod pieces at the bottom of the slow cooker.
Add the reduced sweet potatoes and chopped spinach.
Sprinkle the dill and drizzle the lemon juice on top.

3. Cooking:
Cover the slow cooker with the lid.
Set the slow cooker to low heat and cook for 6-8 hours, or until the cod is fully cooked and the vegetables are tender.

4. Final Touches:
Stir the mixture well to ensure even distribution of ingredients.
Allow to cool before serving.

PORTION CONTROL AND SIZE RECOMMENDATIONS:

Small Dogs (10-20 lbs): 1/2 cup per meal
Medium Dogs (20-50 lbs): 1 cup per meal
Large Dogs (50+ lbs): 1 1/2 - 2 cups per meal

NUTRITIONAL INFORMATION AND CALORIE REQUIREMENTS:

Small Portion (1/2 cup):
Calories: 165 kcal
Protein: 14g
Fat: 6g
Carbohydrates: 9g

Medium Portion (1 cup):
Calories: 330 kcal
Protein: 28g
Fat: 12g
Carbohydrates: 18g

Large Portion (2 cups):
Calories: 660 kcal
Protein: 56g
Fat: 24g
Carbohydrates: 36g

ADAPTATIONS FOR DIFFERENT LIFE STAGES, BREEDS, AND ACTIVITY LEVELS:

Puppies:
Increase protein by adding an extra 1/4 cup of chopped cod.
Ensure the mixture is finely chopped for easier digestion.

Adults:
Follow the standard recipe.

Seniors:
Reduce protein slightly by removing 1/4 cup of cod.
Add an extra 1/4 cup of chopped sweet potatoes for additional fiber.

High-Activity Dogs:
Increase portion size by 25% to meet higher energy needs.

Low-Activity Dogs:
Reduce portion size by 25% to prevent overfeeding.

HEARTY FISH AND BUTTERNUT SQUASH STEW

INGREDIENTS

- 2 pounds of cod (boneless, skinless)
- 1 cup of butternut squash (chopped)
- 1 cup of blueberries
- 2 tablespoons of chia seeds
- 1/2 teaspoon of turmeric

INSTRUCTIONS

1. Preparation:
Wash and chop all vegetables and fruits.
Chop the cod into bite-sized pieces.

2. Layering Ingredients:
Place the cod pieces at the bottom of the slow cooker.
Add the chopped butternut squash, blueberries, and chia seeds.
Sprinkle the turmeric on top.

3. Cooking:
Cover the slow cooker with the lid.
Set the slow cooker to low heat and cook for 6-8 hours, or until the cod is fully cooked and the squash is tender.

4. Final Touches:
Stir the mixture well to ensure even distribution of ingredients.
Allow to cool before serving.

PORTION CONTROL AND SIZE RECOMMENDATIONS:

Small Dogs (10-20 lbs): 1/2 cup per meal
Medium Dogs (20-50 lbs): 1 cup per meal
Large Dogs (50+ lbs): 1 1/2 - 2 cups per meal

NUTRITIONAL INFORMATION AND CALORIE REQUIREMENTS:

Small Portion (1/2 cup):
Calories: 160 kcal
Protein: 14g
Fat: 6g
Carbohydrates: 8g

Medium Portion (1 cup):
Calories: 320 kcal
Protein: 28g
Fat: 12g
Carbohydrates: 16g

Large Portion (2 cups):
Calories: 640 kcal
Protein: 56g
Fat: 24g
Carbohydrates: 32g

ADAPTATIONS FOR DIFFERENT LIFE STAGES, BREEDS, AND ACTIVITY LEVELS:

Puppies:
Increase protein by adding an extra 1/4 cup of chopped cod.
Ensure the mixture is finely chopped for easier digestion.

Adults:
Follow the standard recipe.

Seniors:
Reduce protein slightly by removing 1/4 cup of cod.
Add an extra 1/4 cup of butternut squash for additional fiber.

High-Activity Dogs:
Increase portion size by 25% to meet higher energy needs.

Low-Activity Dogs:
Reduce portion size by 25% to prevent overfeeding.

FISH AND SPINACH DELIGHT

INGREDIENTS

- 2 pounds of salmon (boneless, skinless)
- 1 cup of cauliflower rice
- 1 cup of carrots (chopped)
- 1 cup of spinach (chopped)
- 1/2 teaspoon of thyme

INSTRUCTIONS

1. Preparation:
Wash and chop all vegetables.
Chop the salmon into bite-sized pieces.

2. Layering Ingredients:
Place the salmon pieces at the bottom of the slow cooker.
Add the cauliflower rice, chopped carrots, and spinach.
Sprinkle the thyme on top.

3. Cooking:
Cover the slow cooker with the lid.
Set the slow cooker to low heat and cook for 6-8 hours, or until the salmon is fully cooked and the vegetables are tender.

4. Final Touches:
Stir the mixture well to ensure even distribution of ingredients.
Allow to cool before serving.

PORTION CONTROL AND SIZE RECOMMENDATIONS:

Small Dogs (10-20 lbs): 1/2 cup per meal
Medium Dogs (20-50 lbs): 1 cup per meal
Large Dogs (50+ lbs): 1 1/2 - 2 cups per meal

NUTRITIONAL INFORMATION AND CALORIE REQUIREMENTS:

Small Portion (1/2 cup):
Calories: 165 kcal
Protein: 14g
Fat: 7g
Carbohydrates: 8g

Medium Portion (1 cup):
Calories: 330 kcal
Protein: 28g
Fat: 14g
Carbohydrates: 16g

Large Portion (2 cups):
Calories: 660 kcal
Protein: 56g
Fat: 28g
Carbohydrates: 32g

ADAPTATIONS FOR DIFFERENT LIFE STAGES, BREEDS, AND ACTIVITY LEVELS:

Puppies:
Increase protein by adding an extra 1/4 cup of chopped salmon.
Ensure the mixture is finely chopped for easier digestion.

Adults:
Follow the standard recipe.

Seniors:
Reduce protein slightly by removing 1/4 cup of salmon.
Add an extra 1/4 cup of chopped spinach for additional fiber.

High-Activity Dogs:
Increase portion size by 25% to meet higher energy needs.

Low-Activity Dogs:
Reduce portion size by 25% to prevent overfeeding.

FISH AND GREEN BEAN MEDLEY

INGREDIENTS

- 2 pounds of cod (boneless, skinless)
- 1 cup of green beans (chopped)
- 1 cup of broccoli (chopped)
- 1 tablespoon of coconut oil
- 1/2 teaspoon of basil

INSTRUCTIONS

1. Preparation:
Wash and chop all vegetables.
Chop the cod into bite-sized pieces.

2. Layering Ingredients:
Place the cod pieces at the bottom of the slow cooker.
Add the chopped green beans and broccoli.
Drizzle the coconut oil and sprinkle the basil on top.

3. Cooking:
Cover the slow cooker with the lid.
Set the slow cooker to low heat and cook for 6-8 hours, or until the cod is fully cooked and the vegetables are tender.

4. Final Touches:
Stir the mixture well to ensure even distribution of ingredients.
Allow to cool before serving.

PORTION CONTROL AND SIZE RECOMMENDATIONS:

Small Dogs (10-20 lbs): 1/2 cup per meal
Medium Dogs (20-50 lbs): 1 cup per meal
Large Dogs (50+ lbs): 1 1/2 - 2 cups per meal

NUTRITIONAL INFORMATION AND CALORIE REQUIREMENTS:

Small Portion (1/2 cup):
Calories: 170 kcal
Protein: 15g
Fat: 7g
Carbohydrates: 7g

Medium Portion (1 cup):
Calories: 340 kcal
Protein: 30g
Fat: 14g
Carbohydrates: 14g

Large Portion (2 cups):
Calories: 680 kcal
Protein: 60g
Fat: 28g
Carbohydrates: 28g

ADAPTATIONS FOR DIFFERENT LIFE STAGES, BREEDS, AND ACTIVITY LEVELS:

Puppies:
Increase protein by adding an extra 1/4 cup of chopped cod.
Ensure the mixture is finely chopped for easier digestion.

Adults:
Follow the standard recipe.

Seniors:
Reduce protein slightly by removing 1/4 cup of cod.
Add an extra 1/4 cup of chopped green beans for additional fiber.

High-Activity Dogs:
Increase portion size by 25% to meet higher energy needs.

Low-Activity Dogs:
Reduce portion size by 25% to prevent overfeeding.

FISH, APPLE, AND KALE COMBO

INGREDIENTS

- 2 pounds of salmon (boneless, skinless)
- 1 cup of apples (cored and chopped)
- 1 cup of kale (chopped)
- 1 cup of cauliflower rice
- 1/2 teaspoon of rosemary

INSTRUCTIONS

1. Preparation:
Wash and chop all vegetables and fruits.
Chop the salmon into bite-sized pieces.

2. Layering Ingredients:
Place the salmon pieces at the bottom of the slow cooker.
Add the chopped apples, kale, and cauliflower rice.
Sprinkle the rosemary on top.

3. Cooking:
Cover the slow cooker with the lid.
Set the slow cooker to low heat and cook for 6-8 hours, or until the salmon is fully cooked and the vegetables are tender.

4. Final Touches:
Stir the mixture well to ensure even distribution of ingredients.
Allow to cool before serving.

PORTION CONTROL AND SIZE RECOMMENDATIONS:

Small Dogs (10-20 lbs): 1/2 cup per meal
Medium Dogs (20-50 lbs): 1 cup per meal
Large Dogs (50+ lbs): 1 1/2 - 2 cups per meal

NUTRITIONAL INFORMATION AND CALORIE REQUIREMENTS:

Small Portion (1/2 cup):
Calories: 170 kcal
Protein: 15g
Fat: 7g
Carbohydrates: 8g

Medium Portion (1 cup):
Calories: 340 kcal
Protein: 30g
Fat: 14g
Carbohydrates: 16g

Large Portion (2 cups):
Calories: 680 kcal
Protein: 60g
Fat: 28g
Carbohydrates: 32g

ADAPTATIONS FOR DIFFERENT LIFE STAGES, BREEDS, AND ACTIVITY LEVELS:

Puppies:
Increase protein by adding an extra 1/4 cup of chopped salmon.
Ensure the mixture is finely chopped for easier digestion.

Adults:
Follow the standard recipe.

Seniors:
Reduce protein slightly by removing 1/4 cup of salmon.
Add an extra 1/4 cup of chopped apples for additional fiber.

High-Activity Dogs:
Increase portion size by 25% to meet higher energy needs.

Low-Activity Dogs:
Reduce portion size by 25% to prevent overfeeding.

FISH AND CARROT COMFORT STEW

INGREDIENTS

- 2 pounds of cod (boneless, skinless)
- 1 cup of carrots (chopped)
- 1 cup of green beans (chopped)
- 1 tablespoon of flaxseed oil
- 1/2 teaspoon of oregano

INSTRUCTIONS

1. Preparation:
Wash and chop all vegetables.
Chop the cod into bite-sized pieces.

2. Layering Ingredients:
Place the cod pieces at the bottom of the slow cooker.
Add the chopped carrots and green beans.
Drizzle the flaxseed oil and sprinkle the oregano on top.

3. Cooking:
Cover the slow cooker with the lid.
Set the slow cooker to low heat and cook for 6-8 hours, or until the cod is fully cooked and the vegetables are tender.

4. Final Touches:
Stir the mixture well to ensure even distribution of ingredients.
Allow to cool before serving.

PORTION CONTROL AND SIZE RECOMMENDATIONS:

Small Dogs (10-20 lbs): 1/2 cup per meal
Medium Dogs (20-50 lbs): 1 cup per meal
Large Dogs (50+ lbs): 1 1/2 - 2 cups per meal

NUTRITIONAL INFORMATION AND CALORIE REQUIREMENTS:

Small Portion (1/2 cup):
Calories: 165 kcal
Protein: 14g
Fat: 6g
Carbohydrates: 9g

Medium Portion (1 cup):
Calories: 330 kcal
Protein: 28g
Fat: 12g
Carbohydrates: 18g

Large Portion (2 cups):
Calories: 660 kcal
Protein: 56g
Fat: 24g
Carbohydrates: 36g

ADAPTATIONS FOR DIFFERENT LIFE STAGES, BREEDS, AND ACTIVITY LEVELS:

Puppies:
Increase protein by adding an extra 1/4 cup of chopped cod.
Ensure the mixture is finely chopped for easier digestion.

Adults:
Follow the standard recipe.

Seniors:
Reduce protein slightly by removing 1/4 cup of cod.
Add an extra 1/4 cup of chopped carrots for additional fiber.

High-Activity Dogs:
Increase portion size by 25% to meet higher energy needs.

Low-Activity Dogs:
Reduce portion size by 25% to prevent overfeeding.

Chapter 5
Special Diets and Health Conditions

Allergy-Friendly Meals

CHICKEN AND BUTTERNUT SQUASH MIX

INGREDIENTS 1 POUND OF CHICKEN (DICED)

- 1 cup of butternut squash (peeled and cubed)
- 1 cup of peas (fresh or frozen)
- 2 tablespoons of chia seeds
- 1 teaspoon of dill (chopped)

INSTRUCTIONS

1. Preparation:
Chop the butternut squash and dill.
Dice the chicken if not already prepared.

2. Mixing Ingredients:
In a slow cooker, combine the diced chicken, butternut squash, peas, chia seeds, and dill.
Mix thoroughly until well combined.

3. Cooking:
Cover and cook on low for 6-8 hours or on high for 3-4 hours until the chicken is fully cooked and the squash is tender.

4. Final Touches:
Allow the mixture to cool completely before serving.
Store in an airtight container in the refrigerator.

PORTION CONTROL AND SIZE RECOMMENDATIONS: SMALL DOGS (10-20 LBS): 1/2 CUP PER MEAL

Medium Dogs (20-50 lbs): 1 cup per meal
Large Dogs (50+ lbs): 1 1/2 - 2 cups per meal

NUTRITIONAL INFORMATION AND CALORIE REQUIREMENTS:

Small Portion (1/2 cup):
Calories: 130 kcal
Protein: 12g
Fat: 5g
Carbohydrates: 10g

Medium Portion (1 cup):
Calories: 260 kcal
Protein: 24g
Fat: 10g
Carbohydrates: 20g

Large Portion (2 cups):
Calories: 520 kcal
Protein: 48g
Fat: 20g
Carbohydrates: 40g

ADAPTATIONS FOR DIFFERENT LIFE STAGES, BREEDS, AND ACTIVITY LEVELS:

Puppies:
Increase protein by adding an extra 1/4 cup of diced chicken.
Ensure the mixture is finely chopped for easier chewing and digestion.

Adults:
Follow the standard portion recommendations.

Seniors:
Reduce protein slightly by removing 1/4 cup of diced chicken.
Add an extra 1/4 cup of peas for additional fiber.

High-Activity Dogs:
Increase portion size by 25% to meet higher energy needs.

Low-Activity Dogs:
Reduce portion size by 25% to prevent overfeeding.

TURKEY AND SWEET POTATO COMFORT

INGREDIENTS

- 2 pounds of turkey (ground)
- 2 cups of sweet potatoes (peeled and chopped)
- 1 cup of spinach (chopped)
- 1 teaspoon of parsley (chopped)
- 1/2 teaspoon of turmeric

INSTRUCTIONS

1. Preparation:
Clean and chop the sweet potatoes.
Chop the spinach into small pieces.

2. Layering Ingredients:
Place the ground turkey at the bottom of the slow cooker.
Add the chopped sweet potatoes and spinach on top of the turkey.
Sprinkle the parsley and turmeric evenly over the mixture.

3. Cooking:
Cover the slow cooker with the lid and set it to low heat.
Cook for 6-8 hours on low, or until the turkey is fully cooked and the sweet potatoes are tender.

4. Final Touches:
Stir the mixture well to ensure even distribution of ingredients.
Allow to cool before serving.

PORTION CONTROL AND SIZE RECOMMENDATIONS:

Small Dogs: 1/2 cup per meal
Medium Dogs: 1 cup per meal
Large Dogs: 2 cups per meal

NUTRITIONAL INFORMATION AND CALORIE REQUIREMENTS:

Small Portion (1/2 cup):
Calories: 150 kcal
Protein: 12g
Fat: 6g
Carbohydrates: 10g

Medium Portion (1 cup):
Calories: 300 kcal
Protein: 24g
Fat: 12g
Carbohydrates: 20g

Large Portion (2 cups):
Calories: 600 kcal
Protein: 48g
Fat: 24g
Carbohydrates: 40g

ADAPTATIONS FOR DIFFERENT LIFE STAGES, BREEDS, AND ACTIVITY LEVELS:

Puppies:
Increase protein by adding an extra 1/4 cup of ground turkey.
Ensure the mixture is finely chopped for easier digestion.

Adults:
Follow the standard recipe.

Seniors:
Reduce protein slightly by removing 1/4 cup of ground turkey.
Add an extra 1/4 cup of chopped spinach for additional fiber.

High-Activity Dogs:
Increase portion size by 25% to meet higher energy needs.

Low-Activity Dogs:
Reduce portion size by 25% to prevent overfeeding.

BEEF AND PUMPKIN DELIGHT

INGREDIENTS 1 POUND OF DEEF (GROUND OR DICED)

- 1 cup of pumpkin (pureed or diced)
- 1 cup of kale (chopped)
- 1/2 cup of blueberries
- 1 teaspoon of basil (chopped)

INSTRUCTIONS

1. Preparation:
Chop the kale and basil.
If using fresh pumpkin, peel and dice it. If using canned pumpkin, ensure it is pure pumpkin and not pie filling.

2. Mixing Ingredients:
In a slow cooker, combine the beef, pumpkin, chopped kale, blueberries, and basil.
Mix thoroughly until well combined.

3. Cooking:
Cover and cook on low for 6-8 hours or on high for 3-4 hours until the beef is fully cooked and tender.

4. Final Touches:
Allow the mixture to cool completely before serving.
Store in an airtight container in the refrigerator.

PORTION CONTROL AND SIZE RECOMMENDATIONS: SMALL DOGS (10-20 LBS): 1/2 CUP PER MEAL

Medium Dogs (20-50 lbs): 1 cup per meal
Large Dogs (50+ lbs): 1 1/2 - 2 cups per meal

NUTRITIONAL INFORMATION AND CALORIE REQUIREMENTS:

Small Portion (1/2 cup):
Calories: 120 kcal
Protein: 10g
Fat: 5g
Carbohydrates: 8g

Medium Portion (1 cup):
Calories: 240 kcal
Protein: 20g
Fat: 10g
Carbohydrates: 16g

Large Portion (2 cups):
Calories: 480 kcal
Protein: 40g
Fat: 20g
Carbohydrates: 32g

ADAPTATIONS FOR DIFFERENT LIFE STAGES, BREEDS, AND ACTIVITY LEVELS:

Puppies: Increase protein by adding an extra 1/4 cup of ground beef. Ensure the mixture is finely chopped for easier digestion.

Adults: Follow the standard recipe.

Seniors: Reduce protein slightly by removing 1/4 cup of ground beef. Add an extra 1/4 cup of pumpkin for additional fiber.

High-Activity Dogs: Increase portion size by 25% to meet higher energy needs.

Low-Activity Dogs: Reduce portion size by 25% to prevent overfeeding.

LAMB AND QUINOA ALLERGY-FRIENDLY STEW

INGREDIENTS

- 2 pounds of lean lamb (boneless)
- 1 cup of quinoa (cooked and reduced)
- 1 cup of carrots (chopped)
- 1 cup of green beans (chopped)
- 1 teaspoon of rosemary (dried or fresh)

INSTRUCTIONS

1. Preparation:
Clean and chop the lamb into bite-sized pieces.
Cook the quinoa and reduce its volume.
Chop the carrots and green beans into small pieces.

2. Layering Ingredients:
Place the lamb pieces at the bottom of the slow cooker.
Add the cooked quinoa, chopped carrots, and green beans on top of the lamb.
Sprinkle the rosemary evenly over the mixture.

3. Cooking:
Cover the slow cooker with the lid and set it to low heat.
Cook for 6-8 hours on low, or until the lamb is fully cooked and tender.

4. Final Touches:
Stir the mixture well to ensure even distribution of ingredients.
Allow to cool before serving.

PORTION CONTROL AND SIZE RECOMMENDATIONS:

Small Dogs: 1/2 cup per meal
Medium Dogs: 1 cup per meal
Large Dogs: 2 cups per meal

NUTRITIONAL INFORMATION AND CALORIE REQUIREMENTS:

Small Portion (1/2 cup):
Calories: 180 kcal
Protein: 15g
Fat: 8g
Carbohydrates: 12g

Medium Portion (1 cup):
Calories: 360 kcal
Protein: 30g
Fat: 16g
Carbohydrates: 24g

Large Portion (2 cups):
Calories: 720 kcal
Protein: 60g
Fat: 32g
Carbohydrates: 48g

ADAPTATIONS FOR DIFFERENT LIFE STAGES, BREEDS, AND ACTIVITY LEVELS:

Puppies:
Increase protein by adding an extra 1/4 cup of chopped lamb.
Ensure the mixture is finely chopped for easier digestion.

Adults:
Follow the standard recipe.

Seniors:
Reduce protein slightly by removing 1/4 cup of lamb.
Add an extra 1/4 cup of chopped green beans for additional fiber.

High-Activity Dogs:
Increase portion size by 25% to meet higher energy needs.

Low-Activity Dogs:
Reduce portion size by 25% to prevent overfeeding.

SALMON AND VEGETABLE MEDLEY

INGREDIENTS 1 POUND OF SALMON (COOKED AND FLAKED)

1 cup of green beans (chopped)

1 cup of carrots (chopped)

1 apple (chopped, core removed)

1 teaspoon of thyme (chopped)

INSTRUCTIONS

1. Preparation:
Chop the green beans, carrots, apple, and thyme. Cook and flake the salmon if not already prepared.

2. Mixing Ingredients:
In a slow cooker, combine the flaked salmon, green beans, carrots, apple, and thyme.
Mix thoroughly until well combined.

3. Cooking:
Cover and cook on low for 4-6 hours or on high for 2-3 hours until the vegetables are tender.

4. Final Touches:
Allow the mixture to cool completely before serving.
Store in an airtight container in the refrigerator.

PORTION CONTROL AND SIZE RECOMMENDATIONS: SMALL DOGS (10-20 LBS): 1/2 CUP PER MEAL

Medium Dogs (20-50 lbs): 1 cup per meal
Large Dogs (50+ lbs): 1 1/2 - 2 cups per meal

NUTRITIONAL INFORMATION AND CALORIE REQUIREMENTS:

Small Portion (1/2 cup):
Calories: 110 kcal
Protein: 9g
Fat: 4g
Carbohydrates: 10g

Medium Portion (1 cup):
Calories: 220 kcal
Protein: 18g
Fat: 8g
Carbohydrates: 20g

Large Portion (2 cups):
Calories: 440 kcal
Protein: 36g
Fat: 16g
Carbohydrates: 40g

ADAPTATIONS FOR DIFFERENT LIFE STAGES, BREEDS, AND ACTIVITY LEVELS:

Puppies: Increase protein by adding an extra 1/4 cup of flaked salmon. Ensure the mixture is finely chopped for easier digestion.

Adults: Follow the standard recipe.

Seniors: Reduce protein slightly by removing 1/4 cup of salmon. Add an extra 1/4 cup of chopped green beans for additional fiber. Ensure the mixture is soft enough for older dogs to chew easily.

High-Activity Dogs: Increase portion size by 25% to meet higher energy needs.

Low-Activity Dogs: Reduce portion size by 25% to prevent overfeeding.

LEAN CHICKEN AND VEGETABLE STEW

INGREDIENTS

- 2 pounds of chicken breast (boneless, skinless)
- 1 cup of carrots (chopped)
- 1 cup of green beans (chopped)
- 1 cup of quinoa (cooked)
- 1 teaspoon of parsley (chopped)

INSTRUCTIONS

1. Preparation:
Clean and chop the chicken breast into bite-sized pieces.
Chop the carrots and green beans into small pieces.
Cook the quinoa as per package instructions.

2. Layering Ingredients:
Place the chicken pieces at the bottom of the slow cooker.
Add the chopped carrots, green beans, and cooked quinoa on top of the chicken.
Sprinkle the parsley evenly over the mixture.

3. Cooking:
Cover the slow cooker with the lid.
Set the slow cooker to low heat and cook for 6-8 hours, or until the chicken is fully cooked and tender.

4. Final Touches:
Stir the mixture well to ensure even distribution of ingredients.
Allow to cool before serving.

PORTION CONTROL AND SIZE RECOMMENDATIONS:

Small Dogs: 1/2 cup per meal
Medium Dogs: 1 cup per meal
Large Dogs: 2 cups per meal

NUTRITIONAL INFORMATION AND CALORIE REQUIREMENTS:

Small Portion (1/2 cup):
Calories: 150 kcal
Protein: 18g
Fat: 3g
Carbohydrates: 12g
Medium Portion (1 cup):
Calories: 300 kcal
Protein: 36g
Fat: 6g
Carbohydrates: 24g
Large Portion (2 cups):
Calories: 600 kcal
Protein: 72g
Fat: 12g
Carbohydrates: 48g

ADAPTATIONS FOR DIFFERENT LIFE STAGES, BREEDS, AND ACTIVITY LEVELS:

Puppies:
Increase protein by adding an extra 1/4 cup of chopped chicken.
Ensure the mixture is finely chopped for easier digestion.
Adults:
Follow the standard recipe.
Seniors:
Reduce protein slightly by removing 1/4 cup of chicken.
Add an extra 1/4 cup of chopped green beans for additional fiber.
High-Activity Dogs:
Increase portion size by 25% to meet higher energy needs.
Low-Activity Dogs:
Reduce portion size by 25% to prevent overfeeding.

LIGHT TURKEY AND SPINACH MIX

INGREDIENTS

- 2 pounds of turkey breast (boneless, skinless)
- 1 cup of spinach (chopped)
- 1 cup of sweet potatoes (chopped)
- 1 teaspoon of turmeric
- 1 teaspoon of rosemary (chopped)

INSTRUCTIONS

1. Preparation:
Clean and chop the turkey breast into bite-sized pieces.
Chop the spinach and sweet potatoes into small pieces.

2. Layering Ingredients:
Place the turkey pieces at the bottom of the slow cooker.
Add the chopped spinach and sweet potatoes on top of the turkey.
Sprinkle the turmeric and rosemary evenly over the mixture.

3. Cooking:
Cover the slow cooker with the lid.
Set the slow cooker to low heat and cook for 6-8 hours, or until the turkey is fully cooked and tender.

4. Final Touches:
Stir the mixture well to ensure even distribution of ingredients.
Allow to cool before serving.

PORTION CONTROL AND SIZE RECOMMENDATIONS:

Small Dogs: 1/2 cup per meal
Medium Dogs: 1 cup per meal
Large Dogs: 2 cups per meal

NUTRITIONAL INFORMATION AND CALORIE REQUIREMENTS:

Small Portion (1/2 cup):
Calories: 140 kcal
Protein: 16g
Fat: 4g
Carbohydrates: 10g

Medium Portion (1 cup):
Calories: 280 kcal
Protein: 32g
Fat: 8g
Carbohydrates: 20g

Large Portion (2 cups):
Calories: 560 kcal
Protein: 64g
Fat: 16g
Carbohydrates: 40g

ADAPTATIONS FOR DIFFERENT LIFE STAGES, BREEDS, AND ACTIVITY LEVELS:

Puppies:
Increase protein by adding an extra 1/4 cup of chopped turkey.
Ensure the mixture is finely chopped for easier digestion.

Adults:
Follow the standard recipe.

Seniors:
Reduce protein slightly by removing 1/4 cup of turkey.
Add an extra 1/4 cup of chopped spinach for additional fiber.

High-Activity Dogs:
Increase portion size by 25% to meet higher energy needs.

Low-Activity Dogs:
Reduce portion size by 25% to prevent overfeeding.

LOW-CALORIE BEEF AND PUMPKIN MEDLEY

INGREDIENTS

- 2 pounds of lean beef (ground or cubed)
- 1 cup of pumpkin (cooked and mashed)
- 1 cup of kale (chopped)
- 1/2 cup of blueberries
- 1 teaspoon of basil (chopped)

INSTRUCTIONS

1. Preparation:
Clean and chop the lean beef into bite-sized pieces if using cubed beef.
Cook and mash the pumpkin.
Chop the kale into small pieces.

2. Layering Ingredients:
Place the beef pieces at the bottom of the slow cooker.
Add the mashed pumpkin, chopped kale, and blueberries on top of the beef.
Sprinkle the basil evenly over the mixture.

3. Cooking:
Cover the slow cooker with the lid.
Set the slow cooker to low heat and cook for 6-8 hours, or until the beef is fully cooked and tender.

4. Final Touches:
Stir the mixture well to ensure even distribution of ingredients.
Allow to cool before serving.

PORTION CONTROL AND SIZE RECOMMENDATIONS:

Small Dogs: 1/2 cup per meal
Medium Dogs: 1 cup per meal
Large Dogs: 2 cups per meal

NUTRITIONAL INFORMATION AND CALORIE REQUIREMENTS:

Small Portion (1/2 cup):
Calories: 140 kcal
Protein: 16g
Fat: 5g
Carbohydrates: 8g

Medium Portion (1 cup):
Calories: 280 kcal
Protein: 32g
Fat: 10g
Carbohydrates: 16g

Large Portion (2 cups):
Calories: 560 kcal
Protein: 64g
Fat: 20g
Carbohydrates: 32g

ADAPTATIONS FOR DIFFERENT LIFE STAGES, BREEDS, AND ACTIVITY LEVELS:

Puppies:
Increase protein by adding an extra 1/4 cup of chopped beef.
Ensure the mixture is finely chopped for easier digestion.

Adults:
Follow the standard recipe.

Seniors:
Reduce protein slightly by removing 1/4 cup of beef.
Add an extra 1/4 cup of chopped kale for additional fiber.

High-Activity Dogs:
Increase portion size by 25% to meet higher energy needs.

Low-Activity Dogs:
Reduce portion size by 25% to prevent overfeeding.

TRIM LAMB AND CARROT CASSEROLE

INGREDIENTS

- 2 pounds of lean lamb (cubed)
- 1 cup of carrots (chopped)
- 1 cup of green beans (chopped)
- 1/4 cup of chia seeds
- 1 teaspoon of thyme (chopped)

INSTRUCTIONS

1. Preparation:

Clean and chop the lean lamb into bite-sized pieces.

Chop the carrots and green beans into small pieces.

2. Layering Ingredients:

Place the lamb pieces at the bottom of the slow cooker.

Add the chopped carrots, green beans, and chia seeds on top of the lamb.

Sprinkle the thyme evenly over the mixture.

3. Cooking:

Cover the slow cooker with the lid.

Set the slow cooker to low heat and cook for 6-8 hours, or until the lamb is fully cooked and tender.

4. Final Touches:

Stir the mixture well to ensure even distribution of ingredients.

Allow to cool before serving.

PORTION CONTROL AND SIZE RECOMMENDATIONS:

Small Dogs: 1/2 cup per meal
Medium Dogs: 1 cup per meal
Large Dogs: 2 cups per meal

NUTRITIONAL INFORMATION AND CALORIE REQUIREMENTS:

Small Portion (1/2 cup):
Calories: 150 kcal
Protein: 15g
Fat: 7g
Carbohydrates: 8g

Medium Portion (1 cup):
Calories: 300 kcal
Protein: 30g
Fat: 14g
Carbohydrates: 16g

Large Portion (2 cups):
Calories: 600 kcal
Protein: 60g
Fat: 28g
Carbohydrates: 32g

ADAPTATIONS FOR DIFFERENT LIFE STAGES, BREEDS, AND ACTIVITY LEVELS:

Puppies:
Increase protein by adding an extra 1/4 cup of chopped lamb.
Ensure the mixture is finely chopped for easier digestion.

Adults:
Follow the standard recipe.

Seniors:
Reduce protein slightly by removing 1/4 cup of lamb.
Add an extra 1/4 cup of chopped carrots for additional fiber.

High-Activity Dogs:
Increase portion size by 25% to meet higher energy needs.

Low-Activity Dogs:
Reduce portion size by 25% to prevent overfeeding.

SLIMMING FISH AND BROCCOLI DELIGHT

INGREDIENTS

- 2 pounds of cod
- 1 cup of broccoli (chopped)
- 1 cup of cauliflower rice
- 1 teaspoon of dill
- 1 tablespoon of lemon juice

INSTRUCTIONS

1. Preparation:
Clean and chop the white fish into bite-sized pieces.
Chop the broccoli into small pieces.

2. Layering Ingredients:
Place the fish pieces at the bottom of the slow cooker.
Add the chopped broccoli and cauliflower rice on top of the fish.
Sprinkle the dill and lemon juice evenly over the mixture.

3. Cooking:
Cover the slow cooker with the lid.
Set the slow cooker to low heat and cook for 6-8 hours, or until the fish is fully cooked and tender.

4. Final Touches:
Stir the mixture well to ensure even distribution of ingredients.
Allow to cool before serving.

PORTION CONTROL AND SIZE RECOMMENDATIONS:

Small Dogs: 1/2 cup per meal
Medium Dogs: 1 cup per meal
Large Dogs: 2 cups per meal

NUTRITIONAL INFORMATION AND CALORIE REQUIREMENTS:

Small Portion (1/2 cup):
Calories: 130 kcal
Protein: 18g
Fat: 3g
Carbohydrates: 8g
Medium Portion (1 cup):
Calories: 260 kcal
Protein: 36g
Fat: 6g
Carbohydrates: 16g
Large Portion (2 cups):
Calories: 520 kcal
Protein: 72g
Fat: 12g
Carbohydrates: 32g

ADAPTATIONS FOR DIFFERENT LIFE STAGES, BREEDS, AND ACTIVITY LEVELS:

Puppies:
Increase protein by adding an extra 1/4 cup of chopped fish.
Ensure the mixture is finely chopped for easier digestion.
Adults:
Follow the standard recipe.
Seniors:
Reduce protein slightly by removing 1/4 cup of fish.
Add an extra 1/4 cup of chopped broccoli for additional fiber.
High-Activity Dogs:
Increase portion size by 25% to meet higher energy needs.
Low-Activity Dogs:
Reduce portion size by 25% to prevent overfeeding.

MATURE CHICKEN AND VEGETABLE MEDLEY

INGREDIENTS

- 2 pounds of chicken breast (boneless, skinless)
- 1 cup of cauliflower rice
- 1 cup of zucchini (chopped)
- 1 tablespoon of flaxseed oil
- 1 teaspoon of basil (dried or fresh)

INSTRUCTIONS

1. Preparation:
Clean and cut the chicken breast into bite-sized pieces.
Prepare the cauliflower rice as per package instructions.
Chop the zucchini into small pieces.

2. Layering Ingredients:
Place the chicken pieces at the bottom of the slow cooker.
Add the cauliflower rice and chopped zucchini on top of the chicken.
Drizzle flaxseed oil and sprinkle basil evenly over the mixture.

3. Cooking:
Cover the slow cooker with the lid.
Set the slow cooker to low heat and cook for 6-8 hours, or until the chicken is fully cooked and tender.

4. Final Touches:
Stir the mixture well to ensure even distribution of ingredients.
Allow to cool before serving.

PORTION CONTROL AND SIZE RECOMMENDATIONS:

Small Dogs: 1/2 cup per meal
Medium Dogs: 1 cup per meal
Large Dogs: 2 cups per meal

NUTRITIONAL INFORMATION AND CALORIE REQUIREMENTS:

Small Portion (1/2 cup):
Calories: 130 kcal
Protein: 15g
Fat: 6g
Carbohydrates: 5g
Medium Portion (1 cup):
Calories: 260 kcal
Protein: 30g
Fat: 12g
Carbohydrates: 10g
Large Portion (2 cups):
Calories: 520 kcal
Protein: 60g
Fat: 24g
Carbohydrates: 20g

ADAPTATIONS FOR SPECIFIC LIFE STAGE AND ACTIVITY LEVEL:

Senior Dogs:
Reduce protein slightly by removing 1/4 cup of chicken. Add an extra 1/4 cup of cauliflower rice for additional fiber.
Low-Activity Dogs:
Reduce portion size by 25% to prevent overfeeding.

GOLDEN YEARS TURKEY AND QUINOA MIX

INGREDIENTS

- 2 pounds of turkey breast (boneless, skinless)
- 1 cup of quinoa (cooked and reduced)
- 1 cup of carrots (peeled and diced)
- 1 cup of spinach (chopped)
- 1 teaspoon of rosemary (dried or fresh)

INSTRUCTIONS

1. Preparation:

Clean and cut the turkey breast into bite-sized pieces.
Cook and reduce the quinoa as per package instructions.
Peel and dice the carrots.
Chop the spinach into small pieces.

2. Layering Ingredients:

Place the turkey pieces at the bottom of the slow cooker.
Add the cooked quinoa, diced carrots, and chopped spinach on top of the turkey.
Sprinkle rosemary evenly over the mixture.

3. Cooking:

Cover the slow cooker with the lid.
Set the slow cooker to low heat and cook for 6-8 hours, or until the turkey is fully cooked and the carrots are tender.

4. Final Touches:

Stir the mixture well to ensure even distribution of ingredients.
Allow to cool before serving.

PORTION CONTROL AND SIZE RECOMMENDATIONS:

Small Dogs: 1/2 cup per meal
Medium Dogs: 1 cup per meal
Large Dogs: 2 cups per meal

NUTRITIONAL INFORMATION AND CALORIE REQUIREMENTS:

Small Portion (1/2 cup):
Calories: 130 kcal
Protein: 15g
Fat: 4g
Carbohydrates: 10g
Medium Portion (1 cup):
Calories: 260 kcal
Protein: 30g
Fat: 8g
Carbohydrates: 20g
Large Portion (2 cups):
Calories: 520 kcal
Protein: 60g
Fat: 16g
Carbohydrates: 40g

ADAPTATIONS FOR SPECIFIC LIFE STAGE AND ACTIVITY LEVEL:

Senior Dogs:
Reduce protein slightly by removing 1/4 cup of turkey. Add an extra 1/4 cup of chopped spinach for additional fiber.
Low-Activity Dogs:
Reduce portion size by 25% to prevent overfeeding.

AGING GRACEFULLY BEEF AND BROCCOLI DELIGHT

INGREDIENTS

- 2 pounds of lean beef (ground or cubed)
- 1 cup of broccoli (chopped)
- 1 cup of peas (fresh or frozen)
- 1 teaspoon of parsley (chopped)
- 1 tablespoon of olive oil

INSTRUCTIONS

1. Preparation:

Clean and cut the beef into bite-sized pieces or use ground beef.

Chop the broccoli into small pieces.

If using fresh peas, rinse them thoroughly.

2. Layering Ingredients:

Place the beef at the bottom of the slow cooker.

Add the chopped broccoli and peas on top of the beef.

Sprinkle parsley and drizzle olive oil evenly over the mixture.

3. Cooking:

Cover the slow cooker with the lid.

Set the slow cooker to low heat and cook for 6-8 hours, or until the beef is fully cooked and tender.

4. Final Touches:

Stir the mixture well to ensure even distribution of ingredients.

Allow to cool before serving.

PORTION CONTROL AND SIZE RECOMMENDATIONS:

Small Dogs: 1/2 cup per meal
Medium Dogs: 1 cup per meal
Large Dogs: 2 cups per meal

NUTRITIONAL INFORMATION AND CALORIE REQUIREMENTS:

Small Portion (1/2 cup):
Calories: 150 kcal
Protein: 14g
Fat: 8g
Carbohydrates: 6g

Medium Portion (1 cup):
Calories: 300 kcal
Protein: 28g
Fat: 16g
Carbohydrates: 12g

Large Portion (2 cups):
Calories: 600 kcal
Protein: 56g
Fat: 32g
Carbohydrates: 24g

ADAPTATIONS FOR SPECIFIC LIFE STAGE AND ACTIVITY LEVEL:

Senior Dogs:
Reduce protein slightly by removing 1/4 cup of beef. Add an extra 1/4 cup of chopped broccoli for additional fiber.

Low-Activity Dogs:
Reduce portion size by 25% to prevent overfeeding.

ELDER LAMB AND PUMPKIN FEAST

INGREDIENTS

- 2 pounds of lean lamb (boneless)
- 1 cup of pumpkin (cooked and mashed)
- 1 cup of kale (chopped)
- 1/2 cup of blueberries
- 1 teaspoon of thyme (dried or fresh)

INSTRUCTIONS

1. Preparation:
Clean and chop the lamb into bite-sized pieces.
Cook and mash the pumpkin.
Chop the kale into small pieces.
Rinse the blueberries thoroughly.

2. Layering Ingredients:
Place the lamb pieces at the bottom of the slow cooker.
Add the mashed pumpkin, chopped kale, and blueberries on top of the lamb.
Sprinkle thyme evenly over the mixture.

3. Cooking:
Cover the slow cooker with the lid.
Set the slow cooker to low heat and cook for 6-8 hours, or until the lamb is fully cooked and tender.

4. Final Touches:
Stir the mixture well to ensure even distribution of ingredients.
Allow to cool before serving.

PORTION CONTROL AND SIZE RECOMMENDATIONS:

Small Dogs: 1/2 cup per meal
Medium Dogs: 1 cup per meal
Large Dogs: 2 cups per meal

NUTRITIONAL INFORMATION AND CALORIE REQUIREMENTS:

Small Portion (1/2 cup):
Calories: 140 kcal
Protein: 12g
Fat: 7g
Carbohydrates: 9g

Medium Portion (1 cup):
Calories: 280 kcal
Protein: 24g
Fat: 14g
Carbohydrates: 18g

Large Portion (2 cups):
Calories: 560 kcal
Protein: 48g
Fat: 28g
Carbohydrates: 36g

ADAPTATIONS FOR SPECIFIC LIFE STAGE AND ACTIVITY LEVEL:

Senior Dogs:
Reduce protein slightly by removing 1/4 cup of lamb. Add an extra 1/4 cup of chopped kale for additional fiber.

Low-Activity Dogs:
Reduce portion size by 25% to prevent overfeeding.

SENIOR SALMON AND SWEET POTATO STEW

INGREDIENTS

- 2 pounds of salmon (boneless, skinless)
- 1 cup of sweet potatoes (peeled and diced)
- 1 cup of green beans (chopped)
- 1 teaspoon of turmeric
- 2 tablespoons of chia seeds

INSTRUCTIONS

1. Preparation:

Clean and cut the salmon into bite-sized pieces.
Peel and dice the sweet potatoes.
Chop the green beans into small pieces.

2. Layering Ingredients:

Place the salmon pieces at the bottom of the slow cooker.
Add the diced sweet potatoes and chopped green beans on top of the salmon.
Sprinkle turmeric and chia seeds evenly over the mixture.

3. Cooking:

Cover the slow cooker with the lid.
Set the slow cooker to low heat and cook for 6-8 hours, or until the sweet potatoes are tender and the salmon is fully cooked.

4. Final Touches:

Stir the mixture well to ensure even distribution of ingredients.
Allow to cool before serving.

PORTION CONTROL AND SIZE RECOMMENDATIONS:

Small Dogs: 1/2 cup per meal
Medium Dogs: 1 cup per meal
Large Dogs: 2 cups per meal

NUTRITIONAL INFORMATION AND CALORIE REQUIREMENTS:

Small Portion (1/2 cup):
Calories: 140 kcal
Protein: 14g
Fat: 6g
Carbohydrates: 8g

Medium Portion (1 cup):
Calories: 280 kcal
Protein: 28g
Fat: 12g
Carbohydrates: 16g

Large Portion (2 cups):
Calories: 560 kcal
Protein: 56g
Fat: 24g
Carbohydrates: 32g

ADAPTATIONS FOR SPECIFIC LIFE STAGE AND ACTIVITY LEVEL:

Senior Dogs:
Reduce protein slightly by removing 1/4 cup of salmon. Add an extra 1/4 cup of chopped green beans for additional fiber.

Low-Activity Dogs:
Reduce portion size by 25% to prevent overfeeding.

VEGGIE DELIGHT STEW

INGREDIENTS

- 2 pounds of sweet potatoes (peeled and cubed)
- 1 cup of green beans (chopped)
- 1 cup of carrots (sliced)
- 1 teaspoon of parsley (chopped)
- 2 tablespoons of flaxseed oil

INSTRUCTIONS

1. Preparation:
Peel and cube the sweet potatoes.
Chop the green beans and slice the carrots.
Measure and prepare the parsley and flaxseed oil.

2. Layering Ingredients:
Place the sweet potatoes at the bottom of the slow cooker.
Add the green beans and carrots on top.
Sprinkle the parsley evenly over the vegetables.
Drizzle the flaxseed oil over the mixture.

3. Cooking:
Cover the slow cooker with the lid.
Set the slow cooker to low heat and cook for 6-8 hours, or until the vegetables are tender.

4. Final Touches:
Stir the mixture well to ensure even distribution of ingredients.
Allow to cool before serving.

PORTION CONTROL AND SIZE RECOMMENDATIONS:

Small Dogs: 1/2 cup per meal
Medium Dogs: 1 cup per meal
Large Dogs: 2 cups per meal

NUTRITIONAL INFORMATION AND CALORIE REQUIREMENTS:

Small Portion (1/2 cup):
Calories: 120 kcal
Protein: 2g
Fat: 5g
Carbohydrates: 16g

Medium Portion (1 cup):
Calories: 240 kcal
Protein: 4g
Fat: 10g
Carbohydrates: 32g

Large Portion (2 cups):
Calories: 480 kcal
Protein: 8g
Fat: 20g
Carbohydrates: 64g

ADAPTATIONS FOR DIFFERENT LIFE STAGES, BREEDS, AND ACTIVITY LEVELS:

Puppies:
Increase protein by adding 1/4 cup of cooked lentils.
Ensure the mixture is finely chopped for easier digestion.

Adults:
Follow the standard recipe.

Seniors:
Reduce protein slightly by removing 1/4 cup of sweet potatoes.
Add an extra 1/4 cup of green beans for additional fiber.

High-Activity Dogs:
Increase portion size by 25% to meet higher energy needs.

Low-Activity Dogs:
Reduce portion size by 25% to prevent overfeeding.

HEARTY PUMPKIN AND SPINACH MEDLEY

INGREDIENTS

- 2 pounds of pumpkin (peeled and cubed)
- 1 cup of spinach (chopped)
- 1 cup of quinoa (cooked)
- 1 teaspoon of basil (chopped)
- 2 tablespoons of coconut oil

INSTRUCTIONS

1. Preparation:
Peel and cube the pumpkin.
Chop the spinach.
Cook the quinoa according to package instructions.
Measure and prepare the basil and coconut oil.

2. Layering Ingredients:
Place the pumpkin at the bottom of the slow cooker.
Add the cooked quinoa and chopped spinach on top.
Sprinkle the basil evenly over the mixture.
Drizzle the coconut oil over the ingredients.

3. Cooking:
Cover the slow cooker with the lid.
Set the slow cooker to low heat and cook for 6-8 hours, or until the pumpkin is tender.

4. Final Touches:
Stir the mixture well to ensure even distribution of ingredients.
Allow to cool before serving.

PORTION CONTROL AND SIZE RECOMMENDATIONS:

Small Dogs: 1/2 cup per meal
Medium Dogs: 1 cup per meal
Large Dogs: 2 cups per meal

NUTRITIONAL INFORMATION AND CALORIE REQUIREMENTS:

Small Portion (1/2 cup):
Calories: 110 kcal
Protein: 3g
Fat: 6g
Carbohydrates: 12g
Medium Portion (1 cup):
Calories: 220 kcal
Protein: 6g
Fat: 12g
Carbohydrates: 24g
Large Portion (2 cups):
Calories: 440 kcal
Protein: 12g
Fat: 24g
Carbohydrates: 48g

ADAPTATIONS FOR DIFFERENT LIFE STAGES, BREEDS, AND ACTIVITY LEVELS:

Puppies:
Increase protein by adding 1/4 cup of chopped chicken breast.
Ensure the mixture is finely chopped for easier digestion.
Adults:
Follow the standard recipe.
Seniors:
Reduce protein slightly by removing 1/4 cup of quinoa.
Add an extra 1/4 cup of chopped spinach for additional fiber.
High-Activity Dogs:
Increase portion size by 25% to meet higher energy needs.
Low-Activity Dogs:
Reduce portion size by 25% to prevent overfeeding.

CAULIFLOWER AND KALE CASSEROLE

INGREDIENTS

- 2 pounds of cauliflower rice
- 1 cup of kale (chopped)
- 1 cup of peas (fresh or frozen)
- 1 teaspoon of chia seeds
- 1 teaspoon of rosemary (chopped)

INSTRUCTIONS

1. Preparation:
Prepare the cauliflower rice.
Chop the kale.
Measure and prepare the peas, chia seeds, and rosemary.

2. Layering Ingredients:
Place the cauliflower rice at the bottom of the slow cooker.
Add the peas and chopped kale on top.
Sprinkle the chia seeds and rosemary evenly over the mixture.

3. Cooking:
Cover the slow cooker with the lid.
Set the slow cooker to low heat and cook for 6-8 hours, or until the vegetables are tender.

4. Final Touches:
Stir the mixture well to ensure even distribution of ingredients.
Allow to cool before serving.

PORTION CONTROL AND SIZE RECOMMENDATIONS:

Small Dogs: 1/2 cup per meal
Medium Dogs: 1 cup per meal
Large Dogs: 2 cups per meal

NUTRITIONAL INFORMATION AND CALORIE REQUIREMENTS:

Small Portion (1/2 cup):
Calories: 100 kcal
Protein: 3g
Fat: 2g
Carbohydrates: 18g

Medium Portion (1 cup):
Calories: 200 kcal
Protein: 6g
Fat: 4g
Carbohydrates: 36g

Large Portion (2 cups):
Calories: 400 kcal
Protein: 12g
Fat: 8g
Carbohydrates: 72g

ADAPTATIONS FOR DIFFERENT LIFE STAGES, BREEDS, AND ACTIVITY LEVELS:

Puppies:
Increase protein by adding 1/4 cup of chopped turkey.
Ensure the mixture is finely chopped for easier digestion.

Adults:
Follow the standard recipe.

Seniors:
Reduce protein slightly by removing 1/4 cup of peas.
Add an extra 1/4 cup of kale for additional fiber.

High-Activity Dogs:
Increase portion size by 25% to meet higher energy needs.

Low-Activity Dogs:
Reduce portion size by 25% to prevent overfeeding.

BUTTERNUT SQUASH AND ZUCCHINI MIX

INGREDIENTS

- 2 pounds of butternut squash (peeled and cubed)
- 1 cup of zucchini (chopped)
- 1 teaspoon of turmeric
- 1 cup of green beans (chopped)
- 2 tablespoons of olive oil

INSTRUCTIONS

1. Preparation:
Peel and cube the butternut squash.
Chop the zucchini and green beans.
Measure and prepare the turmeric and olive oil.

2. Layering Ingredients:
Place the butternut squash at the bottom of the slow cooker.
Add the zucchini and green beans on top.
Sprinkle the turmeric evenly over the mixture.
Drizzle the olive oil over the ingredients.

3. Cooking:
Cover the slow cooker with the lid.
Set the slow cooker to low heat and cook for 6-8 hours, or until the squash is tender.

4. Final Touches:
Stir the mixture well to ensure even distribution of ingredients.
Allow to cool before serving.

PORTION CONTROL AND SIZE RECOMMENDATIONS:

Small Dogs: 1/2 cup per meal
Medium Dogs: 1 cup per meal
Large Dogs: 2 cups per meal

NUTRITIONAL INFORMATION AND CALORIE REQUIREMENTS:

Small Portion (1/2 cup):
Calories: 110 kcal
Protein: 2g
Fat: 5g
Carbohydrates: 14g

Medium Portion (1 cup):
Calories: 220 kcal
Protein: 4g
Fat: 10g
Carbohydrates: 28g

Large Portion (2 cups):
Calories: 440 kcal
Protein: 8g
Fat: 20g
Carbohydrates: 56g

ADAPTATIONS FOR DIFFERENT LIFE STAGES, BREEDS, AND ACTIVITY LEVELS:

Puppies:
Increase protein by adding 1/4 cup of chopped chicken.
Ensure the mixture is finely chopped for easier digestion.

Adults:
Follow the standard recipe.

Seniors:
Reduce protein slightly by removing 1/4 cup of butternut squash.
Add an extra 1/4 cup of chopped green beans for additional fiber.

High-Activity Dogs:
Increase portion size by 25% to meet higher energy needs.

Low-Activity Dogs:
Reduce portion size by 25% to prevent overfeeding.

SWEET POTATO AND BROCCOLI FEAST

INGREDIENTS

- 2 pounds of sweet potatoes (peeled and cubed)
- 1 cup of broccoli (chopped)
- 1 cup of carrots (sliced)
- 1 teaspoon of dill (chopped)
- 2 tablespoons of flaxseed oil

INSTRUCTIONS

1. Preparation:
Peel and cube the sweet potatoes.
Chop the broccoli and slice the carrots.
Measure and prepare the dill and flaxseed oil.

2. Layering Ingredients:
Place the sweet potatoes at the bottom of the slow cooker.
Add the broccoli and carrots on top.
Sprinkle the dill evenly over the mixture.
Drizzle the flaxseed oil over the ingredients.

3. Cooking:
Cover the slow cooker with the lid.
Set the slow cooker to low heat and cook for 6-8 hours, or until the vegetables are tender.

4. Final Touches:
Stir the mixture well to ensure even distribution of ingredients.
Allow to cool before serving.

PORTION CONTROL AND SIZE RECOMMENDATIONS:

Small Dogs: 1/2 cup per meal
Medium Dogs: 1 cup per meal
Large Dogs: 2 cups per meal

NUTRITIONAL INFORMATION AND CALORIE REQUIREMENTS:

Small Portion (1/2 cup):
Calories: 120 kcal
Protein: 3g
Fat: 6g
Carbohydrates: 14g

Medium Portion (1 cup):
Calories: 240 kcal
Protein: 6g
Fat: 12g
Carbohydrates: 28g

Large Portion (2 cups):
Calories: 480 kcal
Protein: 12g
Fat: 24g
Carbohydrates: 56g

ADAPTATIONS FOR DIFFERENT LIFE STAGES, BREEDS, AND ACTIVITY LEVELS:

Puppies:
Increase protein by adding 1/4 cup of chopped turkey.
Ensure the mixture is finely chopped for easier digestion.

Adults:
Follow the standard recipe.

Seniors:
Reduce protein slightly by removing 1/4 cup of sweet potatoes.
Add an extra 1/4 cup of chopped broccoli for additional fiber.

High-Activity Dogs:
Increase portion size by 25% to meet higher energy needs.

Low-Activity Dogs:
Reduce portion size by 25% to prevent overfeeding.

Chapter 6
Special Occasion Snacks

How to Incorporate These Recipes

Introducing special occasion snacks into your dog's diet can be a delightful way to celebrate holidays and milestones while ensuring they receive the best nutrition. Designed for events like birthdays, holidays, and festive seasons, these recipes offer more than just a tasty treat. They serve as a practical solution for enhancing your dog's diet with nutrient-rich, vet-approved ingredients.

Special occasion snacks can be seamlessly incorporated into your dog's regular feeding routine without disrupting their nutritional balance. These snacks are made with high-quality proteins, healthy fats, and essential vitamins and minerals, making them both delicious and beneficial for your dog's health. For example, *Holiday Turkey and Cranberry Delight* not only adds a festive flair but also provides antioxidants from cranberries and lean protein from turkey, supporting your dog's overall health.

One of the key benefits of these snacks is their ability to cater to specific dietary needs and preferences. For instance, if your dog has allergies or sensitivities, homemade snacks allow you to avoid common allergens found in commercial treats. Recipes such as *Valentine's Day Chicken* and *Sweet Potato Hearts* can be tailored to exclude ingredients your dog cannot tolerate, ensuring they enjoy their treat without any adverse effects.

By taking advantage of frozen and preserved options, these recipes can be adapted to be enjoyed any time of the year, ensuring your dog always has a nutritious and delicious snack available. The festive names of these recipes are merely indicative; they don't restrict their use to specific times of the year.

Incorporating these snacks into your dog's diet is easy and can be managed alongside their regular meals. Use these treats as rewards for good behavior or during training sessions. Portion control is crucial: for small dogs, limit to 1-2 bites per day; medium dogs can have 3-4 bites, and large dogs 5-6 bites. This ensures they receive the benefits without overeating.

These special snacks also enhance the bond between you and your dog. The act of preparing these treats for yourself shows love and care, strengthening your relationship. Imagine the joy on your dog's face when they get a taste of *Halloween Pumpkin and Carrot Crunchies*, knowing it was made especially for them. This personal touch makes each snack more than just food; it's a token of affection and attention.

Additionally, these homemade snacks are designed to be economical and easy to prepare. Ingredients like sweet potatoes, blueberries, and ground turkey are affordable and readily available, making the preparation process straightforward. Using a slow cooker for batch cooking ensures you can make large quantities with minimal effort, making it perfect for busy owners.

Lastly, these recipes are crafted with the guidance of veterinary nutrition standards, ensuring each treat supports your dog's health. By using ingredients that comply with AAFCO and NRC guidelines, you can be confident that every snack is nutritionally balanced and safe for your dog.

Holiday and Celebration Recipes

BIRTHDAY BEEF AND BLUEBERRY BITES

INGREDIENTS

- 1 pound of lean beef (ground)
- 1/2 cup of blueberries (fresh or frozen)
- 1 cup of oats (gluten-free if necessary)
- 2 large eggs
- 1 tablespoon of parsley (chopped)
- 1 teaspoon of turmeric

INSTRUCTIONS

1. Preparation:
Preheat your slow cooker on low heat.
Combine the ground beef, blueberries, oats, eggs, chopped parsley, and turmeric in a large mixing bowl. Mix thoroughly until well combined.

2. Forming the Biscuits:
Roll the mixture into small bite-sized balls or shape them into small patties.
Place the formed bites in a single layer at the bottom of the slow cooker.

3. Cooking:
Cover the slow cooker with the lid.
Cook on low heat for 6-8 hours or until the bites are fully cooked and firm.

4. Final Touches:
Allow the bites to cool completely before serving.
Store in an airtight container in the refrigerator.

PORTION CONTROL AND SIZE RECOMMENDATIONS:

Small Dogs: 1-2 bites per day
Medium Dogs: 3-4 bites per day
Large Dogs: 5-6 bites per day

NUTRITIONAL INFORMATION AND CALORIE REQUIREMENTS:

Small Portion (1-2 bites):
Calories: 50-100 kcal
Protein: 4-8g
Fat: 2-4g
Carbohydrates: 3-6g
Medium Portion (3-4 bites):
Calories: 150-200 kcal
Protein: 12-16g
Fat: 6-8g
Carbohydrates: 9-12g
Large Portion (5-6 bites):
Calories: 250-300 kcal
Protein: 20-24g
Fat: 10-12g
Carbohydrates: 15-18g

ADAPTATIONS FOR DIFFERENT LIFE STAGES, BREEDS, AND ACTIVITY LEVELS:

Puppies: Increase protein by adding an extra 1/4 cup of ground beef. Ensure the mixture is finely chopped for easier digestion.
Adults: Follow the standard recipe.
Seniors: Reduce protein slightly by removing 1/4 cup of ground beef. Add an extra 1/4 cup of chopped parsley for additional fiber.
High-Activity Dogs: Increase portion size by 25% to meet higher energy needs.
Low-Activity Dogs: Reduce portion size by 25% to prevent overfeeding.

HOLIDAY TURKEY AND CRANBERRY DELIGHTS

INGREDIENTS

- 1 pound of turkey (ground)
- 1/2 cup of cranberries (fresh or dried, unsweetened)
- 1 cup of sweet potatoes (mashed)
- 1 teaspoon of rosemary (chopped)
- 1 tablespoon of flaxseed oil

INSTRUCTIONS

1. Preparation:
Preheat your slow cooker on low heat.
Combine the ground turkey, cranberries, mashed sweet potatoes, chopped rosemary, and flaxseed oil in a large mixing bowl. Mix thoroughly until well combined.

2. Forming the Treats:
Shape the mixture into small patties or rolls. Place the formed treats in a single layer at the bottom of the slow cooker.

3. Cooking:
Cover the slow cooker with the lid.
Cook on low heat for 6-8 hours or until the treats are fully cooked and firm.

4. Final Touches:
Allow the treats to cool completely before serving. Store in an airtight container in the refrigerator.

PORTION CONTROL AND SIZE RECOMMENDATIONS:

Small Dogs: 1-2 treats per day
Medium Dogs: 3-4 treats per day
Large Dogs: 5-6 treats per day

NUTRITIONAL INFORMATION AND CALORIE REQUIREMENTS:

Small Portion (1-2 treats):
Calories: 40-80 kcal
Protein: 3-6g
Fat: 2-4g
Carbohydrates: 2-4g
Medium Portion (3-4 treats):
Calories: 120-160 kcal
Protein: 9-12g
Fat: 6-8g
Carbohydrates: 6-8g
Large Portion (5-6 treats):
Calories: 200-240 kcal
Protein: 15-18g
Fat: 10-12g
Carbohydrates: 10-12g

ADAPTATIONS FOR DIFFERENT LIFE STAGES, BREEDS, AND ACTIVITY LEVELS:

Puppies: Increase protein by adding an extra 1/4 cup of ground turkey. Ensure the mixture is finely chopped for easier digestion.
Adults: Follow the standard recipe.
Seniors: Reduce protein slightly by removing 1/4 cup of ground turkey. Add an extra 1/4 cup of mashed sweet potatoes for additional fiber.
High-Activity Dogs: Increase portion size by 25% to meet higher energy needs.
Low-Activity Dogs: Reduce portion size by 25% to prevent overfeeding.

HALLOWEEN PUMPKIN AND CARROT CRUNCHIES

INGREDIENTS

- 1 cup of pumpkin puree
- 1/2 cup of carrots (grated)
- 1 cup of coconut flour
- 2 large eggs
- 1 teaspoon of ginger

INSTRUCTIONS

1. Preparation:
Preheat your slow cooker on low heat.
Combine the pumpkin puree, grated carrots, coconut flour, eggs, and ginger in a large mixing bowl. Mix thoroughly until well combined.

2. Forming the Crunchies:
Shape the mixture into small balls or patties.
Place the formed crunchies in a single layer at the bottom of the slow cooker.

3. Cooking:
Cover the slow cooker with the lid.
Cook on low heat for 6-8 hours or until the crunchies are firm and fully cooked.

4. Final Touches:
Allow the crunchies to cool completely before serving.
Store in an airtight container in the refrigerator.

PORTION CONTROL AND SIZE RECOMMENDATIONS:

Small Dogs: 1-2 crunchies per day
Medium Dogs: 3-4 crunchies per day
Large Dogs: 5-6 crunchies per day

NUTRITIONAL INFORMATION AND CALORIE REQUIREMENTS:

Small Portion (1-2 crunchies):
Calories: 30-60 kcal
Protein: 1-2g
Fat: 1-2g
Carbohydrates: 3-6g

Medium Portion (3-4 crunchies):
Calories: 90-120 kcal
Protein: 3-4g
Fat: 3-4g
Carbohydrates: 9-12g

Large Portion (5-6 crunchies):
Calories: 150-180 kcal
Protein: 5-6g
Fat: 5-6g
Carbohydrates: 15-18g

ADAPTATIONS FOR DIFFERENT LIFE STAGES, BREEDS, AND ACTIVITY LEVELS:

Puppies:
Increase protein by adding an extra 1/4 cup of grated carrots.
Ensure the mixture is finely chopped for easier digestion.

Adults:
Follow the standard recipe.

Seniors:
Reduce protein slightly by removing 1/4 cup of grated carrots.
Add an extra 1/4 cup of pumpkin puree for additional fiber.

High-Activity Dogs:
Increase portion size by 25% to meet higher energy needs.

Low-Activity Dogs:
Reduce portion size by 25% to prevent overfeeding.

VALENTINE'S DAY CHICKEN AND SWEET POTATO HEARTS

INGREDIENTS

- 1 pound of chicken (ground)
- 1 cup of sweet potatoes (mashed)
- 1/2 cup of applesauce (unsweetened)
- 1 tablespoon of flaxseed meal
- 1 teaspoon of turmeric

INSTRUCTIONS

1. Preparation:
Preheat your slow cooker on low heat.
Combine the ground chicken, mashed sweet potatoes, applesauce, flaxseed meal, and turmeric in a large mixing bowl. Mix thoroughly until well combined.

2. Forming the Hearts:
Shape the mixture into heart-shaped patties using a cookie cutter or by hand.
Place the formed hearts in a single layer at the bottom of the slow cooker.

3. Cooking:
Cover the slow cooker with the lid.
Cook on low heat for 6-8 hours or until the hearts are fully cooked and firm.

4. Final Touches:
Allow the hearts to cool completely before serving.
Store in an airtight container in the refrigerator.

PORTION CONTROL AND SIZE RECOMMENDATIONS:

Small Dogs: 1-2 hearts per day
Medium Dogs: 3-4 hearts per day
Large Dogs: 5-6 hearts per day

NUTRITIONAL INFORMATION AND CALORIE REQUIREMENTS:

Small Portion (1-2 hearts):
Calories: 40-80 kcal
Protein: 4-8g
Fat: 2-4g
Carbohydrates: 3-6g

Medium Portion (3-4 hearts):
Calories: 120-160 kcal
Protein: 12-16g
Fat: 6-8g
Carbohydrates: 9-12g

Large Portion (5-6 hearts):
Calories: 200-240 kcal
Protein: 20-24g
Fat: 10-12g
Carbohydrates: 15-18g

ADAPTATIONS FOR DIFFERENT LIFE STAGES, BREEDS, AND ACTIVITY LEVELS:

Puppies:
Increase protein by adding an extra 1/4 cup of ground chicken.
Ensure the mixture is finely chopped for easier digestion.

Adults:
Follow the standard recipe.

Seniors:
Reduce protein slightly by removing 1/4 cup of ground chicken.
Add an extra 1/4 cup of mashed sweet potatoes for additional fiber.

High-Activity Dogs:
Increase portion size by 25% to meet higher energy needs.

Low-Activity Dogs:
Reduce portion size by 25% to prevent overfeeding.

SUMMER BBQ LAMB AND MINT PATTIES

INGREDIENTS

- 1 pound of lamb (ground)
- 1 tablespoon of fresh mint (chopped)
- 1 cup of quinoa (cooked)
- 1/2 cup of peas (fresh or frozen)
- 1 tablespoon of coconut oil
- 1 teaspoon of ginger

INSTRUCTIONS

1. Preparation:
Preheat your slow cooker on low heat.
Combine the ground lamb, chopped mint, cooked quinoa, peas, coconut oil, and ginger in a large mixing bowl. Mix thoroughly until well combined.

2. Forming the Patties:
Shape the mixture into small patties.
Place the formed patties in a single layer at the bottom of the slow cooker.

3. Cooking:
Cover the slow cooker with the lid.
Cook on low heat for 6-8 hours or until the patties are fully cooked and firm.

4. Final Touches:
Allow the patties to cool completely before serving.
Store in an airtight container in the refrigerator.

PORTION CONTROL AND SIZE RECOMMENDATIONS:

Small Dogs: 1-2 patties per day
Medium Dogs: 3-4 patties per day
Large Dogs: 5-6 patties per day

NUTRITIONAL INFORMATION AND CALORIE REQUIREMENTS:

Small Portion (1-2 patties):
Calories: 50-100 kcal
Protein: 5-10g
Fat: 3-6g
Carbohydrates: 2-4g

Medium Portion (3-4 patties):
Calories: 150-200 kcal
Protein: 15-20g
Fat: 9-12g
Carbohydrates: 6-8g

Large Portion (5-6 patties):
Calories: 250-300 kcal
Protein: 25-30g
Fat: 15-18g
Carbohydrates: 10-12g

ADAPTATIONS FOR DIFFERENT LIFE STAGES, BREEDS, AND ACTIVITY LEVELS:

Puppies:
Increase protein by adding an extra 1/4 cup of ground lamb.
Ensure the mixture is finely chopped for easier digestion.

Adults:
Follow the standard recipe.

Seniors:
Reduce protein slightly by removing 1/4 cup of ground lamb.
Add an extra 1/4 cup of quinoa for additional fiber.

High-Activity Dogs:
Increase portion size by 25% to meet higher energy needs.

Low-Activity Dogs:
Reduce portion size by 25% to prevent overfeeding.

SPRINGTIME CHICKEN AND PEA BLOSSOMS

INGREDIENTS

- 1 cup of chicken (cooked and chopped)
- 1 cup of peas (fresh or frozen)
- 1 cup of quinoa
- 1 cup of carrots (chopped)
- 1 teaspoon of basil

INSTRUCTIONS

1. Preparation:
Cook and chop the chicken.
Rinse the quinoa.
2. Layering Ingredients:
Place chicken, peas, quinoa, and carrots in the slow cooker.
Add basil.
3. Cooking:
Cover the slow cooker with the lid.
Set to low heat and cook for 4-6 hours, or until the mixture is firm and well combined.
4. Final Touches:
Stir the mixture well.
Allow to cool before shaping into flower-shaped blossoms.

PORTION CONTROL AND SIZE RECOMMENDATIONS:

Small Dogs: 1-2 blossoms per treat
Medium Dogs: 2-4 blossoms per treat
Large Dogs: 4-6 blossoms per treat

NUTRITIONAL INFORMATION AND CALORIE REQUIREMENTS:

Small Portion (1-2 blossoms):
Calories: 35 kcal
Protein: 3g
Fat: 1g
Carbohydrates: 4g
Medium Portion (2-4 blossoms):
Calories: 70 kcal
Protein: 6g
Fat: 2g
Carbohydrates: 8g
Large Portion (4-6 blossoms):
Calories: 105 kcal
Protein: 9g
Fat: 3g
Carbohydrates: 12g

ADAPTATIONS FOR DIFFERENT LIFE STAGES, BREEDS, AND ACTIVITY LEVELS:

Puppies:
Ensure the blossoms are small and soft for easier chewing.
Increase protein by adding an extra 1/4 cup of cooked chicken.
Adults:
Follow the standard recipe.
Seniors:
Make sure the blossoms are soft enough for older dogs to chew easily.
Reduce protein slightly by removing 1/4 cup of cooked chicken.
High-Activity Dogs:
Increase portion size by 25% to meet higher energy needs.
Low-Activity Dogs:
Reduce portion size by 25% to prevent overfeeding.

AUTUMN APPLE AND CARROT NIBBLES

INGREDIENTS

- 2 cups of carrots (chopped)
- 2 apples (cored and chopped)
- 1 cup of oats (gluten-free if necessary)
- 2 tablespoons of chia seeds
- 2 tablespoons of honey
- 1 teaspoon of turmeric

INSTRUCTIONS

1. Preparation:
Wash and chop the carrots and apples.
Combine the chopped carrots, apples, oats, chia seeds, honey, and turmeric in a large mixing bowl.
Mix thoroughly until well combined.

2. Layering Ingredients:
Transfer the mixture to the slow cooker, ensuring even layer.

3. Cooking:
Set the slow cooker to low and cook for 4-5 hours, stirring occasionally, until the ingredients are soft and well blended.

4. Final Touches:
Allow the mixture to cool completely before serving.
Store in an airtight container in the refrigerator.

PORTION CONTROL AND SIZE RECOMMENDATIONS:

Small Dogs (10-20 lbs): 1/4 cup per meal
Medium Dogs (20-50 lbs): 1/2 cup per meal
Large Dogs (50+ lbs): 3/4 - 1 cup per meal

NUTRITIONAL INFORMATION AND CALORIE REQUIREMENTS:

Small Portion (1/4 cup):
Calories: 50 kcal
Protein: 1g
Fat: 2g
Carbohydrates: 10g

Medium Portion (1/2 cup):
Calories: 100 kcal
Protein: 2g
Fat: 4g
Carbohydrates: 20g

Large Portion (3/4 - 1 cup):
Calories: 150-200 kcal
Protein: 3-4g
Fat: 6-8g
Carbohydrates: 30-40g

ADAPTATIONS FOR DIFFERENT LIFE STAGES, BREEDS, AND ACTIVITY LEVELS:

Puppies:
Ensure the mixture is finely chopped for easier chewing and digestion.
Increase protein by adding an extra 1/4 cup of chopped carrots.

Adults:
Follow the standard portion recommendations.

Seniors:
Make sure the mixture is soft enough for older dogs to chew easily.
Reduce protein slightly by removing 1/4 cup of chopped carrots.

High-Activity Dogs:
Increase portion size by 25% to meet higher energy needs.

Low-Activity Dogs:
Reduce portion size by 25% to prevent overfeeding.

FOURTH OF JULY SALMON AND SPINACH STARS

INGREDIENTS

- 1 cup of salmon (cooked and flaked)
- 1 cup of spinach (chopped)
- 1 cup of brown rice flour
- 2 eggs
- 1 teaspoon of turmeric

INSTRUCTIONS

1. Preparation:
Cook and flake the salmon.
Chop the spinach.

2. Layering Ingredients:
Place salmon and spinach in the slow cooker.
Add brown rice flour, eggs, and turmeric.

3. Cooking:
Cover the slow cooker with the lid.
Set to low heat and cook for 4-6 hours, or until the mixture is firm and well combined.

4. Final Touches:
Stir the mixture well.
Allow to cool before shaping into star-shaped treats.

PORTION CONTROL AND SIZE RECOMMENDATIONS:

Small Dogs: 1-2 stars per treat
Medium Dogs: 2-4 stars per treat
Large Dogs: 4-6 stars per treat

NUTRITIONAL INFORMATION AND CALORIE REQUIREMENTS:

Small Portion (1-2 stars):
Calories: 40 kcal
Protein: 4g
Fat: 1.5g
Carbohydrates: 3g

Medium Portion (2-4 stars):
Calories: 80 kcal
Protein: 8g
Fat: 3g
Carbohydrates: 6g

Large Portion (4-6 stars):
Calories: 120 kcal
Protein: 12g
Fat: 4.5g
Carbohydrates: 9g

ADAPTATIONS FOR DIFFERENT LIFE STAGES, BREEDS, AND ACTIVITY LEVELS:

Puppies:
Ensure the stars are small and soft for easier chewing.
Increase protein by adding an extra 1/4 cup of cooked salmon.

Adults:
Follow the standard recipe.

Seniors:
Make sure the stars are soft enough for older dogs to chew easily.
Reduce protein slightly by removing 1/4 cup of cooked salmon.

High-Activity Dogs:
Increase portion size by 25% to meet higher energy needs.

Low-Activity Dogs:
Reduce portion size by 25% to prevent overfeeding.

NEW YEAR'S EVE CHICKEN AND BUTTERNUT SQUASH MUNCHIES

INGREDIENTS 1 POUND OF CHICKEN (CUBED OR SHREDDED)

- 1 cup of butternut squash (peeled and cubed)
- 1 cup of carrots (chopped)
- 1 tablespoon of chia seeds
- 1 teaspoon of parsley (chopped)

INSTRUCTIONS

1. Preparation:
Wash and chop all vegetables.
Cut the chicken into cubes or shred it.

2. Layering Ingredients:
Place the cubed chicken, butternut squash, carrots, chia seeds, and parsley in a slow cooker.

3. Cooking:
Set the slow cooker to low and cook for 6-8 hours or until the chicken is fully cooked and the vegetables are tender.

4. Final Touches:
Allow the mixture to cool completely before serving.
Store in an airtight container in the refrigerator.

PORTION CONTROL AND SIZE RECOMMENDATIONS: SMALL DOGS (10-20 LBS): 1/2 CUP PER MEAL

Medium Dogs (20-50 lbs): 1 cup per meal
Large Dogs (50+ lbs): 1 1/2 - 2 cups per meal

NUTRITIONAL INFORMATION AND CALORIE REQUIREMENTS:

Small Portion (1/2 cup):
Calories: 90 kcal
Protein: 10g
Fat: 2g
Carbohydrates: 8g

Medium Portion (1 cup):
Calories: 180 kcal
Protein: 20g
Fat: 4g
Carbohydrates: 16g

Large Portion (2 cups):
Calories: 360 kcal
Protein: 40g
Fat: 8g
Carbohydrates: 32g

ADAPTATIONS FOR DIFFERENT LIFE STAGES, BREEDS, AND ACTIVITY LEVELS:

Puppies:
Ensure the mixture is finely chopped for easier chewing and digestion.
Increase protein by adding an extra 1/4 cup of diced chicken.

Adults:
Follow the standard portion recommendations.

Seniors:
Make sure the mixture is soft enough for older dogs to chew easily.
Reduce protein slightly by removing 1/4 cup of diced chicken.

High-Activity Dogs:
Increase portion size by 25% to meet higher energy needs.

Low-Activity Dogs:
Reduce portion size by 25% to prevent overfeeding.

CHRISTMAS TURKEY AND QUINOA SNOWBALLS

INGREDIENTS

- 1 cup of turkey (cooked and chopped)
- 1 cup of quinoa
- 1 cup of kale (chopped)
- 1 cup of apples (cored and chopped)
- 1 teaspoon of turmeric

INSTRUCTIONS

1. Preparation:
Cook and chop the turkey.
Rinse the quinoa.
Chop the kale and apples.

2. Layering Ingredients:
Place turkey, quinoa, kale, and apples in the slow cooker.
Add turmeric.

3. Cooking:
Cover the slow cooker with the lid.
Set to low heat and cook for 4-6 hours, or until the mixture is firm and well combined.

4. Final Touches:
Stir the mixture well.
Allow to cool before shaping into snowballs.

PORTION CONTROL AND SIZE RECOMMENDATIONS:

Small Dogs: 1-2 snowballs per treat
Medium Dogs: 2-4 snowballs per treat
Large Dogs: 4-6 snowballs per treat

NUTRITIONAL INFORMATION AND CALORIE REQUIREMENTS:

Small Portion (1-2 snowballs):
Calories: 40 kcal
Protein: 4g
Fat: 1.5g
Carbohydrates: 3g

Medium Portion (2-4 snowballs):
Calories: 80 kcal
Protein: 8g
Fat: 3g
Carbohydrates: 6g

Large Portion (4-6 snowballs):
Calories: 120 kcal
Protein: 12g
Fat: 4.5g
Carbohydrates: 9g

ADAPTATIONS FOR DIFFERENT LIFE STAGES, BREEDS, AND ACTIVITY LEVELS:

Puppies:
Ensure the snowballs are small and soft for easier chewing.
Increase protein by adding an extra 1/4 cup of cooked turkey.

Adults:
Follow the standard recipe.

Seniors:
Make sure the snowballs are soft enough for older dogs to chew easily.
Reduce protein slightly by removing 1/4 cup of cooked turkey.

High-Activity Dogs:
Increase portion size by 25% to meet higher energy needs.

Low-Activity Dogs:
Reduce portion size by 25% to prevent overfeeding.

Chapter 7
Time-Saving and Budget-Friendly Tips

Smart Strategies for Ingredient Management

Providing your dog with nutritious, home-cooked meals on a weekly basis can be rewarding but time-consuming. However, with the appropriate strategies, you may speed up the process, saving time and money while feeding your pet nutritional foods. Therefore, to make the most of your efforts, utilize these simple ideas and practices for smart meal planning, wise food purchases, and leftover repurposing.

A well-organized dog diet relies on effective meal preparation. Firstly, begin with a weekly meal plan that specifies each meal and contains a variety of meats, veggies, and grains. Planning ahead of time not only lowers last-minute stress but also allows you to buy with greater purpose and efficiency.

As a result, careful ingredient selection is a key component of successful meal preparation. Furthermore, to save money on ingredients, buy them in bulk whenever possible. Look for special deals and discounts on premium proteins, vegetables, and grains. Choose inexpensive yet nutritious foods such as poultry, meat, and seasonal veggies. Farmers' markets can provide a great deal of fresh, locally grown produce at affordable prices.

Also, consider purchasing frozen vegetables, which are typically less expensive and equally nutritious as fresh vegetables, allowing you to maintain a diversified kitchen all year. When shopping in bulk, it is critical to properly store fruit to maintain freshness. Purchase airtight containers for cereals and dry items, and vacuum seal meat and veggies. This in turn extends the shelf life of products and guarantees that you always have what you need on hand, preventing frequent shopping trips.

In addition, repurposing leftovers is a creative and cost-effective way to augment the dog's diet while decreasing food waste. You can turn many kitchen scraps and leftovers into nutritious dog food and kibble. For example, you can shred leftover cooked chicken and put it into a vegetable stew, or combine mashed sweet potatoes and oats to make healthy treats. Moreover, add natural supplements to your dog's food to improve his health.

These clever methods and ingredient management tips will ensure that your dog's diet is varied and balanced while saving time and money. Efficient meal planning, budgeting, and repurposing leftovers are all practical methods to make home cooking for your dog more realistic and enjoyable. Your dog will benefit from nutritious, home-cooked meals, and you will have peace of mind knowing exactly what he is eating.

Batch Cooking, Freezing, and Storing

Incorporating batch cooking into your routine saves time and reduces everyday stress by ensuring that your dog always has nutritious meals available. You can ensure your dog's constant supply of nutritious meals by dedicating a few hours every week to preparing huge amounts of food. Therefore, to significantly reduce cooking time, chop up vegetables and divide out proteins ahead of time.

Furthermore, if you have more than one slow cooker, you can cook multiple items at once with minimal oversight; otherwise, stagger cooking durations, beginning with longer recipes like *Lamb and Lentil Soup*. Moreover, if you want to maximize your cooking efforts, opt for meals like *Chicken and Sweet Potato Delight* or *Beef and Spinach Delight*, which are simple to double or triple. Bulk snacks, such *as Sweet Potato and Spinach* (*Delicious Rewards* bonus) can provide your dog with nutritious options in between meals. This technique not only saves time, but also offers peace of mind knowing that you are following a well-planned and consistent diet.

Afterward, divide the food into portion-sized containers according to your dog's dietary needs. To keep track of what you have and use it in time, label each one with the recipe and date before storing it in the freezer. Freezing food preserves its freshness and nutritional value, as well as saving you valuable time. Therefore, invest in high-quality, resealable containers or bags suitable for freezing to keep food fresh and healthy. Let prepared meals cool completely before freezing them to avoid the formation of condensation and ice crystals, which can compromise texture and taste.

Additionally, invest in high-quality, resealable containers or freezer bags to keep food fresh and healthy. Allow prepared meals to cool completely before freezing to minimize condensation and ice crystals, which can degrade texture and flavor. Before storing meals, portion them based on the dog's daily needs. This enables you to defrost just what you need, reducing waste while keeping the food fresh. For increased convenience, thaw meals in the refrigerator overnight or in the microwave. However, to prevent bacterial growth, do not thaw at room temperature.

Moreover, to make your dog's diet more interesting, combine recipes such as *Chicken and Mango Delight* and *Beef and Sweet Potato Delight*. Cook cereals and vegetables slightly undercooked before freezing; they will continue to cook when reheated, preserving their texture and nutritional value. Freezing herbs like parsley or basil in small amounts can enhance the flavor of foods without requiring additional seasoning when warmed.

Enhancing Meals with Supplements

Safe Herbs and Natural Additives

By including natural supplements in your dog's diet, you can guarantee that he or she gets all of the necessary nutrients. Fish oil, flaxseed oil, and chia seeds provide omega-3 fatty acids, which aid in heart health, reduce inflammation, and the development of a lustrous coat. You can incorporate them by mixing a small amount of oil with your dog's meal several times a week.

Additionally, probiotics found in yogurt, kefir, and powdered probiotics improve digestion and immunity. A tablespoon of plain, unsweetened yogurt in your dog's meal promotes digestive health. Meat and bone broth include glucosamine and chondroitin, which are necessary for joint health, particularly in senior dogs. They add flavor and nutrients. Moreover, blueberries, spinach, and sweet potatoes include antioxidants such as vitamins C and E, which help to counteract oxidative stress and promote health. Mixing these into meals improves nutrition and variety.

Including healthful herbs in your dog's food provides several benefits. Turmeric contains strong antioxidant and anti-inflammatory properties that promote joint health and digestion. To improve absorption, mix it with black pepper and some good fat, like coconut oil. Parsley, which contains vitamins A, C, and K, can aid to improve your dog's breath. Simply sprinkle finely chopped parsley over your dog's food or mix it with homemade treats.

Ginger helps with stomach problems by easing nausea and promoting digestion. For instance, including a tiny amount of freshly grated ginger in meals is especially useful for dogs with sensitive stomachs. Rosemary is a natural preservative with antimicrobial characteristics that can improve cognitive function, making it suitable for elderly dogs. Sprinkle dried rosemary over food or use fresh rosemary in slow-cooked meals.

Introducing these nutrients and herbs into your dog's food is straightforward. Start by introducing one vitamin or herb at a time and watching your dog's reaction. Gradually increase the dose to your desired level. Begin with a small amount of fish oil, yogurt, or bone broth and gradually increase it until your dog's system responds adequately.

Moreover, batch cooking is an effective way to include these vitamins and herbs. Prepare large amounts of food, making sure that each meal has an adequate amount of these nutritious additives. A spoonful of fish oil, a sprinkle of turmeric, and some fresh parsley can enhance a slow-cooked chicken, sweet potato, and spinach recipe. This technique ensures your dog receives a variety of nutrients on a consistent basis.

In addition, it is useful to freeze meals containing these vitamins and herbs. To ensure proper absorption, incorporate the herbs and supplements into the food before freezing. Add temperature-sensitive supplements like probiotics or omega-3 oils to the food while it's heating to maintain their effectiveness.

In short, all of these supplements not only give essential nutrients but also contribute to a varied and appetizing diet, making mealtime enjoyable and healthy for your dog. Therefore, before introducing new supplements, visit your veterinarian to confirm they are suitable for your dog's individual health needs.

Unlock Your Exclusive Bonuses!

Thank you for making it this far! I hope you've enjoyed and found the contents of this book practical and beneficial for your furry friend's nutrition. To download the exclusive bonuses I've promised, please email me at **yourbooks.bonuses@gmail.com**

Here are the bonuses you will have access to with the purchase of *Slow Cooker Dog Food Cookbook*:

- **Pawfect Bowls**. Simplify meal planning with a flexible, vet-approved weekly and monthly plan that suits your busy lifestyle.
- **Delicious Rewards**. Delight your furry friend with healthy, easy-to-prepare kibble that complements a balanced diet and training regime.
- **Golden Kitchen**. Complement the main recipe book with another time-saving, effective cooking method that enriches your dog's meals with nutritious, home-cooked goodness for greater health and happiness.
- **Healthy Swaps**. Safely address dietary restrictions with tailored ingredient substitutions that maintain nutritional balance and variety.
- **Dog Diet Dos and Don'ts**. Ensure the safety and well-being of your dog with increased awareness of safe foods and toxic traps.

Thank you once again for your trust and commitment to your dog's health. Happy cooking!

Morgan J. Nichols

Made in the USA
Las Vegas, NV
16 October 2024

96903956R00063